Mary dale
De Bor
860 248 9854

Praise for
A Return to Healing

"Change is in the air for America's health care system. Amid the myriad proposals, the vision expressed in *A Return to Healing* stands out as exceptional—wise, workable, and utterly necessary to steer us from a disease-care model to an authentic, genuine, health care approach. Dr. Len Saputo knows from his experience as a physician that our current system is in many ways unjust, immoral, and shameful. His proposal for integral-health medicine deserves our sincerest consideration. Written in clear, personal language, this book will provide anyone with the information they need to think intelligently about the transitions in health care that will soon affect everyone in America."

—Larry Dossey, MD
Author of *The Power of Premonitions* and *Reinventing Medicine*

"Len Saputo, MD, and co-author Byron Belitsos offer an honest and radically refreshing new strategy for reform that goes beyond the good intentions of whole-person healing, and exposes the hard facts about the flagrant profit-driven agendas within private insurance companies and the medical-pharma-industrial complex. As a clinician, Saputo has worked out the nuts and bolts of integrative practice, and knows firsthand what it takes to keep patients well. His recommendations for transforming our current disease-centric, crumbling paradigm are brilliant, life-saving, and should be immediately adopted by the current administration."

—Meg Jordan, PhD, RN
Department Chair, Integrative Health Studies
California Institute of Integral Studies

"A remarkable book by a remarkable physician. Dr. Saputo offers insider insights into the practice and the politics of medicine as he gives us a prescription that can bring us healing as individuals and as a culture. If you've wondered what's wrong with medicine, and how to fix it, this book should be on your reading list."

—Martin L. Rossman, MD
Author of *Guided Imagery for Self-Healing*

"At last, here is a book about health care that asks the right questions—not *how* can we pay for medical treatment for all, but *what* treatment should we pay for; not *which* drugs should be used first, but *should* drugs be the first line of defense? Len Saputo, MD, writes from his own experience, and he writes very well—clearly, cogently, and in a way that makes you want to keep reading. For a profession burdened with dry medical statistics and not known for its compelling writers, that in itself is an outstanding achievement; but Dr. Saputo does more than just hold your attention. He actually provides much-needed answers to those burning health care questions currently in the news and before Congress. How can we provide health care for the whole population without bankrupting the system? The soaring cost of health care is one of the most formidable aspects of America's financial 'perfect storm,' one that I explore in my own work. Dr. Saputo's solution to this apparently unsolvable problem involves a Copernican shift in our thinking. This book is a must-read for anyone exploring the politics and future of health care."

—Ellen Hodgson Brown, JD
Author of *The Web of Debt* and *Forbidden Medicine*

"This is a story that needed to be told—and who better than a seasoned physician like Len who is so well versed in complementary medicine. We all know and share the frustrations of modern health care in America, but Dr. Saputo opens our eyes to so much more—and then he opens our hearts to real and practical solutions. Joining leaders like President Obama, Saputo is opening the door to positive change at a time when it is most needed. Bravo!"

—Francesco Garri Garripoli
Author of *Qigong: Essence of the Healing Dance*
President of the Qigong Institute

"I highly recommend this inspiring book, both for health care professionals and anyone concerned with our broken system. Len Saputo's experience with 'disease-care' medicine as described in this book matches my own. Health care reform that embraces an integrative model, focuses on prevention, and institutes single-payer insurance is a must—an imperative—if we are to truly transform the state of medicine in this country."

—Stacia Lansman, MD
Founder of Pediatric Alternatives, Mill Valley CA

A Return to Healing

A Return to Healing

Radical Health Care Reform and the Future of Medicine

Len Saputo, MD

with **Byron Belitsos**

ORIGIN PRESS

Origin Press

PO Box 151117 • San Rafael, CA 94915
888.267.4446 • originpress.com

Cover and interior design by theBookDesigners I bookdesigners.com

First printing May 2009

    Saputo, Len.
       A return to healing : radical health care reform and
    the future of medicine / by Len Saputo ; with Byron
    Belitsos.
       p. cm.
       Includes bibliographical references and index.
       LCCN 2009925014
       ISBN-13: 978-1-57983-052-6
       ISBN-10: 1-57983-052-8

       1. Integrative medicine. 2. Holistic medicine.
    3. Health care reform--United States. 4. Medical care--
    United States.   I. Belitsos, Byron, 1953- II. Title.

    R733.S28 2009   610
               QBI09-600039

10 9 8 7 6 5 4 3 2 1

Printed in the United States of America

Contents

Dedication   xv

Acknowledgments   xvii

About the Author   xix

Foreword   xxi

Preface   xxv

Introduction   1

1. A Surprise Healing of My Wife's Illness   9

2. How I Became Part of the Problem: 25
    The Story of My Medical Training

3. How "Scientific" Is Scientific Medicine?   47

4. How Well Is America's Health Care System Working?   87

5. The Karma of Big Pharma: Questioning the Drug Industry   111

6. Wellness, Prevention, and Healing: 139
    The New Direction for Medicine

7. The Birth of the Health Medicine Movement   159

8. Creating an Integrative Medical Clinic   191

9. The Imperative of Radical Health Care Reform   211

Epilogue: The Spirit of Healing   245

Endnotes   249

Bibliography   263

Index   267

Expanded Table of Contents

Dedication   xv

Acknowledgments   xvii

About the Author   xix

Foreword   xxi

Preface   xxv

Introduction   1

Chapter 1
A Surprise Healing of My Wife's Illness   9

Synchronicity comes to Vicki's rescue   12

A turning point in my relationship to medicine   15

I learn a key premise of the new medical paradigm   17

Nature has always done the healing   18

Resistance against the new medicine   19

Getting back to the basics of health   21

We must treat the whole person   23

Chapter 2
How I Became Part of the Problem:
The Story of My Medical Training   25

Len will grow up to be a doctor!   26

True medicine is about healing—isn't it?   29

Medical school may be hazardous to your health   29

Being a clinician is about becoming increasingly human   31

Humility is a central quality of excellence in medicine   33

A startling case of my own depersonalization in medical training   34

More depersonalization in working with live patients   36

The theme of separation is at the heart of the medical model   38

Preparing to be a research scientist at the NIH   39

Severe sleep deprivation and medical postgraduate training   40

Learning how to heal through inspiration, not intimidation   43

Initiating change in medicine through political action   44

Can physicians have their own union today?   45

Chapter 3
How "Scientific" Is Scientific Medicine?   47

My hospital rejects the science of clinical nutrition   50

A hospital pharmacy blocks an essential and   56
scientifically proven nutrient

I face resistance in bringing forward a proven technology   59

Just how evidence based is today's medicine?   65

Ethics issues for research scientists and the FDA   69

Competing scientific models for defining disease   72
and determining treatment

Cellular health: a key concept underlying the new   74
science of medicine

The imperative of properly nourishing our bodies   74

The imperative of detoxification in the face   78
of chemical exposures

Genetic defects disturb cellular biochemistry   81

Our internal pharmacology is regulated by our   81
thoughts and feelings

Modern medicine is at war with nature   82

The failure of our war against diseases   85

Chapter 4
How Well Is America's Health Care System Working?   87

Our increased spending correlates with a   89
chronic-disease epidemic

Just how counterproductive is mainstream medicine?   93

A health care system at the breaking point   97

Hospitals, HMOs, and the central role of   100
the insurance industry

Physicians are discontented with today's medical practice   102

Physicians as well have human needs   104

The acute problems of private health insurance   105

The sad consequence of market-driven health care   107

Chapter 5
The Karma of Big Pharma:
Questioning the Drug Industry   111

The impact of direct-to-consumer drug ads   113

Do you still want to take the purple pill?   117

There's a pill for everything! Or so says Big Pharma   120

Pharmaceutical company ties to Congress   122

Pharmaceutical company ties to physicians   124

Pharmaceutical company ties to medical institutions   127

Big Pharma's bottom line: patent or no patent?   129

Pharma creates a new category: the "worried well"   131

Chapter 6
Wellness, Prevention, and Healing:
The New Direction for Medicine   139

Getting acquainted with the wellness buffer   140

The Pete Wilson and Tim Russert stories   143

Differentiating curing and healing   147

Focusing on the whole person is nearly impossible   148
in the current model

Public surveys reveal what Americans want from medicine   151

Patients and their families demand integrative care   153

The urgent need for birthing a new   156
paradigm of medicine

Chapter 7
The Birth of the Health Medicine Movement   159

Groping for an institutional model for Health Medicine   161

The Health Medicine Forum is born   164

The evolution of the core principles of Health Medicine   167

Integrative practice: the first core principle   169
of Health Medicine

Holism (and integralism): the second core   174
principle of Health Medicine

Person-centered care: the third core principle   179
of Health Medicine

Person-centered care: the beliefs of the patient   180
and the placebo effect

Person-centered care: harvesting the lessons of illness   184

Prevention and wellness: the fourth core   186
principle of Health Medicine

Chapter 8
Creating an Integrative Medical Clinic 191

Practical challenges in our first integrative clinic 194

Starting over with an improved clinical model 197

Healing Circles: a key innovation 198

How Healing Circles work in practice 200

Practitioner responses to Healing Circles 204

Can mainstream and CAM practitioners work together? 207

Chapter 9
The Imperative of Radical Health Care Reform 211

A last look at the health care cost catastrophe 215

The moral problem with private health insurance 216

The economic argument for universal health care 218

Universal health insurance: a crucial debate of our time 221

Physicians favor a single-payer system 222

Creating health and wellness through national 223
prevention policies

Integrative health care and federal health policy 231

Radical reform of the FDA is urgently needed 234

Making medical freedom a constitutional right 237

Revisiting freedom of choice and "evidence-based" medicine 239

The ultimate front line of health care: profit versus service 241

Epilogue: The Spirit of Healing 245
Endnotes 249
Bibliography 263
Index 267

Dedication

*This book is dedicated to my wife, Vicki Saputo.
It speaks of our life's work together over the past 29 years.
My contributions—and this book—would not have
been possible without her sacrifice, insight,
commitment, and love.*

*Thank you, Vicki.
You are my soul mate.*

Acknowledgments

Literally hundreds of people have contributed to the content of this book, and only a few are mentioned by name. Each of you knows who you are, and I believe you will forgive me for not specifically acknowledging your name and contribution. This work is a collective effort and a continuing process that is only in its early stages of development. The Health Medicine movement, which is now evolving into an even more futuristic model that we call *integral medicine* or *integral-health medicine* in this book, promises to be an exciting part of a larger process in the transformation of our social and cultural values.

About the Author

L en Saputo, MD, a 1965 graduate of Duke University Medical School, is board certified in internal medicine and was in private practice in affiliation with John Muir Medical Center in the San Francisco Bay Area for more than 30 years. Len's awakening to the deep flaws in conventional medicine culminated in the early 1990s, propelling him into a quest to develop a new approach to healing. This approach is now known as *integral-health medicine*—the emergent medical care model that is integrative, holistic, person-centered, and preventive.

In order to further this mission, Len founded the Health Medicine Forum in 1994 and was its director until 2008. The Forum (healthmedicineforum.org) is a nonprofit educational foundation that has sponsored hundreds of public and professional events in the San Francisco Bay Area—including monthly presentations, workshops, and conferences—focused on integrative medicine, the nature of healing, and the politics of health care. In 2001, Len cofounded what is now called the Health Medicine Center (healthmedicinecenter.net), in Walnut Creek, California—one of the first clinics to bring the new model of integral-health medicine into practice. In the course of disseminating his unique vision for the new medicine, Len has given more than 100 presentations to hospitals, medical schools, universities, and community organizations.

Len is the coauthor of *Boosting Immunity: Creating Wellness Naturally* (New World Library, 2002); has edited six books, including *Beating the Years* and *Boosting Your Digestive Health*; and has authored book chapters on numerous medical and health subjects. He has contributed dozens of articles on a wide range of topics in both mainstream and complementary and alternative medicine to such journals as *California Pharmacist*, *Alternative Medicine*, and *Townsend Letter*. He is also actively engaged in clinical research related to the use of near-infrared light therapy in pain management.

Active in public and professional education over the past decade, Len produces and hosts the *Prescriptions for Health* show on KEST-AM, aired in the San Francisco Bay Area every weekday morning, with his wife, Vicki, who is a registered nurse.

Len has been a strong advocate of fitness and athletics all of his life. In 1996 and again in 2001, he won the International Tennis Federation's Senior World Individual Championship in his age group and was ranked number one in the world in 1996 (in the 55-year-old division) by the ITF. With never-ending support from his wife, Len is committed to his life's purpose of changing the health care system in America from a disease care model to a genuine health care model based on the principles of the new medicine, as well as broad-ranging reform of the manner in which care is financed and delivered.

Foreword

We've witnessed a revolution in scientific medicine over the past century. Enormous technical achievements can be heralded, from advances in public health to the recent advances in molecular biology, neuroscience, biomedical engineering, and pharmacology. Of course, Americans know that not all the changes have been good. Indeed, there are many indications that medicine is in deep crisis, as Dr. Len Saputo—a long-practicing internal medicine physician—so clearly explains in this important book. Tragically, millions of Americans are without medical coverage. Meanwhile, the costs associated with health care continue to spiral upward, making it harder and harder for people to get the help they need. Iatrogenic (medically induced) illness, Len points out, is another significant challenge, as a result of the large number of new treatments, resistant strains of microbes, and the work overload of many health professionals. Economic pressures reduce the amount of time clinicians can spend with patients, which also contributes to burnout among many on the front lines. These and the many other issues lucidly outlined in *A Return to Healing* point directly to the systematic changes in the medicine model and in America's health care system that Dr. Saputo recommends.

Again, not one of us would dispute the idea that science and technology have resulted in vastly improved understanding, diagnosis, and treatment of disease. But the emphasis on this factor to the exclusion of other elements of healing has also served to limit the development of a model that *humanizes* the health care encounter. Far too often, modern medicine ignores the importance of the personal and interpersonal dimensions of healing and health. Compassion is rarely a selection criterion for medical training, and developing a bedside manner is not featured in the core curriculum of most academic health care programs. As we read the eye-opening story of his own training at Duke University Medical Center in the 1960s, we learn that Len was among those who were taught to avoid or suppress the emotions that are connected to states of disease and healing—both the patient's and the physician's. Over his decades of practice since then, he was witness to the fact that, for patients and professionals alike, the biomedical model too often fails to offer a system that embraces the vast potentials of healing; he shows in fact how this attitude ignores or negates completely the possibility for human growth in the face of illness.

Dr. Saputo's frontline experience with these flaws in the old medical model directly led to his courageous and pioneering crusade for change. These efforts of his, to which I am an appreciative witness, began with his founding of the Health Medicine Forum in 1994, which has transformed the work of thousands of health care practitioners in the San Francisco Bay Area. It has culminated in his founding of an integrative clinic responsible for a number of innovations in integrative methodology, and now in this, his newest book.

Thanks to efforts like those of Len Saputo and many other conventionally trained health professionals who have opened themselves to a new worldview, a fresh breeze is now blowing through many corridors of our hospitals and clinics. Patients and clinicians alike are demanding that the heart and soul of healing be reinstated. There are many positive developments that speak to an emerging new model for health care—one that acknowledges multiple dimensions of living, healing, and curing—dimensions that go beyond a mere reduction of symptoms.

One name for this new model is *integral health care*. Len draws on the same body of emerging theory in this book, calling the new model *integral-health medicine*.

The integral model is based on an intuitive understanding of life and reality as an undivided whole. One of the first modern attempts to bring an integral approach to health care was advanced more than 20 years ago in a book entitled *Mind, Body & Health: Toward an Integral Medicine*, edited by James Gordon, Dennis Jaffe, and David Bresler (Human Sciences Press, 1984). Speaking to the many challenges of Western medicine at that time, they noted that integral-medicine physicians were rediscovering the healing potentials of the patient–physician relationship. Being concerned with the whole person rather than the disease, the authors called on physicians to consider the possibility of a life force that is manifested mentally, physically, and spiritually, and that is the ground of human development and healing.

Now in the 21st century, several new books and conferences have helped to fuel the development of this integral model. An important voice is that of integral philosopher Ken Wilber, who has applied his ideas to the field of health care. Developing a quadrant system, he maps the lines and levels of integral philosophy to include both inner and outer experience, and private and public spheres of exchange. In *Consciousness and Healing: Integral Approaches to Mind Body Medicine*, my colleagues and I explore the same integral terrain as it relates to health and healing through various forms of expression. Contributions by more than 65 authors represent both the depth and the breadth of this emergent field, including the personal and the collective aspects of health and healing. Saputo's vast store of experiences with the medical system and with thousands of patients, as summarized in this book, puts meat on the bones of these more theoretical discussions.

Following in the same territory, Saputo points out that both patients and clinicians comprise psychological, social, cultural, biological, and transpersonal dimensions, which can come together in meaningful synergy in the context of health care and the creation of optimal healing environments.

An integral perspective is as much about healing as it is about curing, he also explains. Just as a health care practitioner might work to mobilize patients' antibodies to fight disease, integral health care involves in equal measure harnessing a patient's desire for health and the will to live. From the integral perspective, these qualitative domains are as significant as the role of scientific information and technology. Finally, in addition to the science of diagnosing, treating, or preventing disease and damage to the body or mind, this is a model that seeks to heal—even in the face of potential death and dying.

Ultimately, the integral perspective calls for a whole-system shift from a disease-centered to a healing-centered model for health care. As Dr. Saputo and his cowriter Byron Belitsos so compelling argue in this inspiring book, it is now time for such a return to healing in America's health care regime.

Marilyn Mandala Schlitz, PhD
President, Institute of Noetic Sciences

Preface

Over the 40 years that I have been in medical practice, I've watched with increasing dismay as commercial values have overtaken mainstream medicine, almost obliterating the central mission of our profession. I have grieved as I have witnessed how the quality of health care in the United States has plunged so far as to be rated among the lowest levels in the developed world.

I entered the profession aspiring to be a healer, as did most of my colleagues. We wanted to attend to the health and medical needs of *whole persons*; we were inspired to serve our patients through our aspiration to provide genuine healing and to promote healthy living based on science and common sense. Sadly, this ideal has been replaced by the corporate bottom line, resulting in a dysfunctional system focused almost entirely on what I prefer to call *disease care*. The physician's natural focus on the health needs of a unique, living person embedded in his family and society has today been largely replaced by a model that reduces each person to his body, his body to a machine, and his health needs to a set of symptoms to be treated mainly with drugs—too often ignoring the patient's mind, emotions, spirit, environment, and lifestyle.

Underlying this shift, and at the heart of the problem, is a culture that accepts—and in fact generates—this reductionistic and mechanistic model of health, along with the costly health care system that has grown up around it. Especially with the rise of for-profit *managed care* in the last three decades and the increasing predominance of a pharmaceutical industry and large hospital chains ever in search of profit, our often counterproductive health care system has become entrenched, even as ordinary Americans have become sicker. The ultimate result is that the heart and soul of true medicine is being lost, left behind in a crazy-quilt system that largely treats symptoms for profit. Meanwhile, Americans are apparently paying more money—much more money—to become less healthy.

But fortunately for you and me, it doesn't have to be this way.

It is heartbreaking to be a practicing physician at a time when the medical system itself has become a leading cause of death and when far too many people are sick in all age groups. It distresses me to watch as "Big Pharma" corporations, impersonal insurance companies, and overpaid HMO (health maintenance organization) bureaucrats have created a Frankenstein system that is no longer affordable for ordinary Americans. It pains me to observe how their allies in government can't or won't regulate them properly, and how they have so far failed to come up with a national health insurance model that works for all Americans. It is heartrending to see so many millions of Americans going without any medical care coverage at all. More of concern to me is the realization that single-payer national insurance—even a system as progressive as those in Canada, the UK, or France—is a necessity but is still not a sufficient solution. National health care reform that is built around the old disease care model of medicine may reduce some costs but will not in the end create much better health for Americans.

But again, it doesn't have to be this way.

We're all in this boat together—all of us are more or less complicit in a system that simply does not work. This is true even of the patients themselves, too many of whom suffer quiescently as they pay the price both in their pocketbooks and in their deteriorating health. At the other end of the scale, our top medical and science professionals are also becoming part of the problem: Serious conflict of interest is rife in research medicine, a fact well documented to exist even at its highest levels—in universities, regulatory agencies, and prestigious medical journals.

Indeed, even today's average doctor can be part of the problem: For although physicians can and do celebrate the fact that the medical technology and basic research they use daily have advanced greatly, any doctor who has practiced over the last several decades will have witnessed a steady deterioration of the general state of medical practice, both in the quality of care that doctors are able to provide to patients and in the satisfactions levels they experience in practicing medicine. Nevertheless, doctors are not yet sufficiently organized to speak out for substantive change.

However, once again, it doesn't have to be this way.

So with all these issues at hand, what's the core problem? Along with many other observers, I believe the central flaw is that business and economics now dominate the industry; what was once the practice of healing based on the precepts of Hippocrates has turned into a business commodity that doles out standardized "treatments" dictated by the requirements of profit. This dominion of business values over our health care, combined with medicine's obsessive attention to treating symptoms rather than to prevention and genuine healing, has led to a general crisis in the health status of Americans—indeed, an epidemic of chronic diseases such as obesity, diabetes, heart disease, and cancer. It has also produced an unaffordable health care delivery system that is threatening the very solvency of the American government. And underlying it all are cultural values that seem to anchor us in alienation, the profit motive, competition, and mechanistic thinking that puts us at war with nature herself.

Also reaching a high point of crisis is the *allopathic* medical paradigm itself, which in this book I usually call the "reductionist," "fundamentalist," "mainstream," or "disease care" model. This approach is at its best in treating acute conditions, and at its worst when promoting health and prevention. But even where it was once strongest, allopathic medicine is now in decline because of its compromised science and its flawed systems of delivery. Knowing this to be true by their own experience, tens of millions of patients are voting against mainstream medicine with their feet, many abandoning it almost entirely.

The old reductionistic model is losing ground to natural medicine and *holistic* or *integrative* methods of healing or treating disease. It is giving way to preventive medicine, new patient-centered models of practice, and the abiding quest for peak lifetime health by millions of thoughtful Americans. The new medicine promotes mind-body-spirit wellness in a way that shifts our focus from *disease* care to genuine *health* care. It recognizes that at the deepest level, physical disease is usually the somatic expression of psychospiritual dysfunction—and that our psychospiritual problems are, in turn, deeply rooted in a society and culture that are themselves generating a systemic, global crisis of survival.

When the many limitations resulting from medicine's mechanistic worldview are combined with the phenomenon of the over-commercialization of the medical industry—its domination by the bottom line and corporations that sometimes literally get away with murder—the result is often outrage, especially from patients and doctors. This book reflects that outrage and then harnesses it toward the mission of a return to healing, including a revival of the desire of physicians, nurses, and health practitioners of every kind to provide high-quality and affordable service.

Carrying out this mission requires a futuristic model of medicine, as proposed in this book—one that is based on my own 40 years of experience plus that of hundreds of colleagues with whom I have been working for over 15 years in my Health Medicine

Forums. This new approach begins with the increasing acceptance of alternative healing methods, leads gradually toward the model of integrative medicine—or what I call *Health Medicine*—and culminates in genuinely *integral medicine*, or the more descriptive phrase I prefer: *integral-health medicine*. Getting there will require the grassroots-driven resolve of the American people for structural change—indeed, the radical reform of health care at every level, including single-payer national insurance for all Americans. It will also require a new understanding of the role of consciousness in healing and a massive public education program that will lead all of us to take full responsibility for our health—to take the lead in medicine away from business and even from well-meaning physicians who are stuck in the system, and put it in the hands of the patients themselves.

After all, it is *your* life that is at stake!

In this book, you will discover how we have come to this great impasse. You will learn how we can turn the medical industry around with a genuine return to healing, led by the desire to serve the true needs of the patient as well as through the readiness of each of us to pursue peak health throughout our own lives. In the end, a return to healing can result only from the rise of a life-affirming global culture that is based on the thrill of serving others—one that sustains and celebrates vibrant health and actively promotes the quest for spiritual progress.

Len Saputo, MD
with Byron Belitsos
Orinda, California
March 2009

Introduction

Just about everyone knows that America's health care system is in deep trouble. Too many people are ill, too many medical treatments are dangerous and even deadly, and basic health care is unaffordable for a large portion of the population. Despite the much-vaunted invasion of health care by "market efficiencies" in the last few decades, the system is nonetheless approaching economic disaster.

The evidence is all around us: As medical costs continue to skyrocket each year, our health care system—if we can even call it a system—has now become the leading cause of personal bankruptcy. Health care costs now consume 18 percent of the gross domestic product (GDP)—two to three times as much as that of comparable nations—even while the quality of care is declining when compared with these same countries.

In fact, the medical care system in the United States does not perform like other businesses in the modern world, which must adapt to meet individual needs and preferences with increasing efficiency. Instead, today's managed care is increasingly impersonal and standardized, is frustrating to most patients and physicians, and relies more than ever on expensive drugs of questionable value.

It has also become clear that we cannot unconditionally trust medical research, the pharmaceutical industry, or even the FDA to set the standards that guide our physicians to create the treatment strategies by which we live or die. As I show in this book, even the supposition that medicine is always based on solid science is simply not true.

It was 30 years ago that renowned sociologist Ivan Illich published *Medical Nemesis*, a prescient indictment of modern medicine, which, he wrote, had itself "become a major threat to health." Today the problems posed by our medical-industrial-pharmaceutical-government complex loom far larger than Illich's original readers could have ever imagined.

Good medicine is so much more than today's mainstream practice of treating a set of disease symptoms with a bag of tools and drugs just to make a profit. Americans want *all* of their health needs met—physical, mental, emotional, and spiritual—and at an affordable cost. And our physicians and healers want a system of delivery that fulfills their desire to provide great medical care and to truly serve their patients. In the opening two chapters of this book, I explain how my own awakening to these fundamental values at midcareer set me on a journey to undo the fallacies of my medical training at Duke University.

My own story is emblematic of a health care system now at the tipping point of a paradigm shift. Massive change is afoot, and this is why the health care crisis is such a hot topic in today's news, and why, especially in chapters 3–5, I intensively reexamine the economics, the politics, and even the basic philosophy of what health care is and how it should be delivered. There can be no doubt about it: We need to face the shortcomings of our health care system and adapt, or there will be even more dire consequences. All stakeholders need to take a much more active role in cocreating a health care paradigm that will meet all of our health needs—and we need to do it *now*.

But unless there is a dramatic shift in the attitude of our conventional medical establishment, such solutions are not likely to come from either our physicians or the medical industry that supports them. There is a common misperception that too much is at stake—financially, professionally, personally, and politically—to put genuine service before the profit motive. Change has been held in check by powerful forces that depend on the status quo for their survival and by the premise—usually unconscious or just below the surface—that "authority" and "precedent" should not be questioned.

But as we stated in the preface, even larger forces are at work: The roots of America's health care crisis have originated not only in the health care system itself but in our dysfunctional cultural values. All of us are responsible for our part, but the grave problems in today's health care are not solely the failure of our physicians, the medical industry, insurance companies, or even our political system. In this book, I identify the true culprit: an underlying fatal fundamentalism, or materialistic reductionism, underpinning how all of society thinks and operates. We have inherited an unhealthy culture that is robotically anchored in separatism, mechanism, isolationism, and fierce competition. It pits us against one another, against the needs of society, and even against the entire universe. It narcissistically supports the concept of "the survival of the fittest." Tragically, this dysfunctional stance embodies the antithesis of what I believe is our intended meaningful purpose in life—to live with peak health and highest happiness in true community.

It will become apparent as this book progresses that it is impossible to fully mend our ailing health care system without implementing a value system in our larger society that honors service before profit and community before narcissistic needs. Of course, one part of this larger cultural and social transformation will be the work of identifying the basic essentials of what is needed to provide good health care. Such a task will require not only the collaborative participation and support of patients, physicians, and the entire health care industry, but also substantive input from political thinkers, spiritual leaders, and philosophers. This process begins with a willingness to reassess the conventionally accepted definition of good health and, once a new model of health care is in hand, a determination to develop creative ways to deliver and pay for it. In chapters 6–8, I describe what I believe to be the emerging new model and narrate the story of my own efforts to discover this new approach in the company of scores of colleagues, as well as my efforts to bring our discoveries into clinical practice.

We can say this much in an introduction: Contrary to mainstream medicine's definition, good health is far more than "the absence of disease."

Yet we do little to estimate our level of wellness, even though we have sophisticated tests that can assess the functional reserves of our body; sadly, these tests are generally given only to the sick. Our bodies are truly amazing in that each organ system has a reserve of about 50 percent more than is necessary to maintain normal function. If we lose more than this reserve, however, our bodies begin to fall apart. When this happens, it is often too late to restore normal function, and we end up with a chronic disability.

But such calamities need not happen today. We know precisely what it takes for nearly every child and adult to have superb health; there's an enormous database of scientific studies verifying that we can support wellness through maintenance of a healthy lifestyle and describing exactly how we can do so at each stage of life. For example, medical science has documented that the precursor for the epidemic of chronic diseases we are now facing is *chronic inflammation*, and we also know that living a healthy lifestyle is the ideal way to prevent inflammation.

It is possible to avoid—through health education from an early age, preventive medicine, and the consistent cultivation of healthy lifestyle factors—the entire panoply of diseases that afflict Americans today, such as cancer, heart disease, strokes, infections, hypertension, diabetes, and autoimmune diseases. We all understand that "an ounce of prevention is worth a pound of cure." It is far easier to prevent disease than to treat it once "the horse is out of the barn." Yet, given our dysfunctional cultural values, we simply cannot find the will to do the obvious.

Ignoring these commonsense practices and relying on medical intervention when sickness occurs is precisely how the bulk of mainstream medicine operates—and consequently, perfecting this approach is what most Americans have been taught is the gold standard for a good health care system.

We all know that the high cost of this style of health care has become a serious financial challenge for patients, businesses, and even the government, and the final chapter of this book examines what to do at the level of national policy. In our misguided fight against disease, 50 percent of all health care costs is spent on terminal illnesses during the last year of life, and yet at the same time, modern medicine believes it does not have the "luxury" of adequately tending to the psychospiritual needs of patients or the promotion of healthy lifestyle practices. Instead, managed care pressures physicians to treat diseases rather than human beings; after all, time is money, and given the high cost of high-tech medicine, there simply isn't sufficient money to pay for more than the bare minimum required to get people on their feet and back to work.

The responsibility of a healer, however, does not end with providing properly functioning biochemistry and physiology—or what I call in this book the act of simply *curing* disease. Curing is merely the process whereby true healing often starts. I show especially in chapter 6 how healing is a much deeper process that uncovers the role of underlying illness, not only in relation to physical ailments and a given set of psychological challenges, but also in the context of the patient's entire life story. These answers are usually buried deeply within, and they often take great wisdom to identify and seasoned skill to resolve.

Historically, ancient healing traditions assigned to the *shaman* the responsibility for guiding patients through life's challenges at all levels. But with the advent of Newtonian science and mechanistic materialism as our dominant mode of thinking, mind and spirit were banished from the practice of medicine and relegated to the domain of religion and the Church. Now, with the advent of quantum mechanics and subsequent discoveries about the physical universe and the nature of human consciousness, scientists are returning to the realization that science and spirituality have always been inseparable. It is becoming clear that our lives are deeply interwoven not only within our community, but also with the entire universe. We are all part of a vast cosmic collective and inseparable whole, and our minds and hearts are linked with minds and hearts everywhere. I further explore some of these ideas throughout the book and in the epilogue.

One of the major goals of this book is to urge you to look deeper into the causes of our failing health care system. I believe you will find that these same causes are expressed in the fatal fundamentalism that plagues *every* aspect of our culture, whether it be health care, business, politics, law, government, or religion. Before we can heal our health care system, we must heal our culture, and we cannot heal our culture unless we are first willing to heal ourselves.

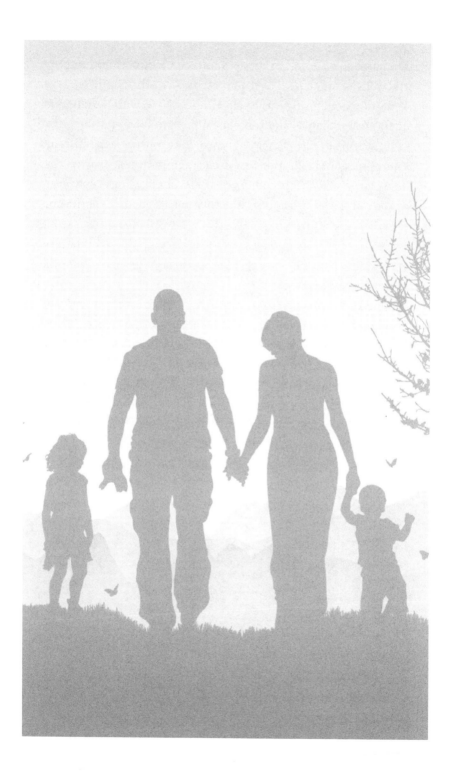

One

A Surprise Healing of My Wife's Illness

Drugs never cure disease. They merely hush the voice of nature's protest, and pull down the danger signals she erects along the pathway of transgression.

—Daniel H. Kress, MD

On the last evening of our vacation to the Orient in October 1991, my wife, Vicki, and I enjoyed a beautiful gourmet dinner by candlelight at the elegant Shangri-La Hotel overlooking the spectacular Hong Kong harbor. Vicki liked her salad so much that she ordered a second. As we returned to our hotel room to pack for the long trip home to San Francisco, the palms of Vicki's hands and the soles of her feet suddenly began to itch. Within minutes she was covered with huge hives, her eyes began burning, her hands and feet began to swell, and her tongue swelled so much that her speech became slurred. We quickly realized that Vicki was exhibiting very serious symptoms of what is known as an anaphylactic allergic reaction.

But this wasn't her first such reaction by any means. In fact, over the previous two years, Vicki had suffered from many severe systemic allergic reactions, which were in each case treated with large doses of two powerful antihistamines, Atarax and Seldane. In dealing with this malady in the past, she and I felt that we knew what we were doing—I being a Duke University–trained MD and Vicki a registered nurse. However, the reaction we were now witnessing in Hong Kong was by far the worst ever, and both of us were terrified. After a few more minutes she fainted, and I could barely detect a pulse.

We were in real trouble—alone on the cold bathroom floor in a hotel in Hong Kong without desperately needed medical supplies. I'll never forget the helpless feeling of being stranded from the tools of my profession and watching my beloved wife rapidly deteriorate. I frantically raced to the hotel telephone and at the same time pleaded with God to let there be a hotel nurse on duty late at night who had access to an emergency drug kit with injectable Adrenalin.

Thank you, God! They had a hotel nurse! I was quickly connected to her.

"Do you have a drug kit with Adrenalin?" I anxiously shouted into the phone.

She responded, "I do, but it is only for emergencies."

"This *is* an emergency," I screamed, "and please hurry!"

As I hung up the phone, there was a knock at the door. I rushed to open it, hoping that somehow the nurse had magically managed to get there instantly, only to see that it was the delivery service from Tommy Lee's Clothing with the shirts, suits, and shoes we'd ordered earlier in the week. "Not now!" I yelled and rushed back to Vicki's side. In all this chaos, the nurse arrived, and I immediately administered the life-saving injection of Adrenalin and an antihistamine. Vicki began to stir.

But we were not out of danger. As the nurse was gathering her supplies in preparation to leave, Vicki's symptoms began to recur. She was having a second anaphylactic attack. After a second injection of Adrenalin, the allergic reaction came under control.

Taking no chances, I then gave her a large oral dose of a powerful steroid called Prednisone to further ensure that the severe allergic reaction would not recur. I wondered if it was the second helping of salad that had caused this entire episode.

We were finally out of immediate danger, but this had been my wife's 23rd anaphylactic reaction, and they were getting worse.

We didn't sleep much that night, not knowing whether another reaction might occur. When Vicki got up to go to the bathroom later, her feet were so swollen that she said it felt like she was walking on inner tubes. I had never been more worried about her.

Vicki had previously been evaluated by the best allergists in our home community in the San Francisco Bay Area. In fact, her allergist was nothing short of wonderful. He was so concerned and caring that he presented her story at Stanford Medical Center's Immunology Grand Rounds. Vicki had undergone every possible relevant test offered by conventional medicine, and the results kept coming back "normal." The final consensus was that she was one of about 25 known cases in medical literature with a disorder called *primary anaphylaxis.* Put simply, this meant that no one knew why she was having recurring anaphylactic reactions, and the best and only treatment option in conventional medicine was to suppress her symptoms with long-term use of steroids, antihistamines, and H2 blockers (another family of drugs that block allergic reactions). We certainly did not want her to have another potentially life-threatening attack, so we reluctantly complied with the treatment program for fear that the next allergic reaction might be fatal.

Thankfully, at the outset, the program worked. However, after a few months of this treatment, Vicki began to have serious side effects. She developed the "moon face" so characteristic of people on Prednisone, and suffered from indigestion, emotional ups and downs, an ankle fracture after only minimal trauma, and irritable bowel syndrome. It appeared that the side effects of the treatment might be as dangerous as the illness. Yet her allergists insisted that she might be on these drugs for the rest of her life. At that point, we knew there were no safe, effective solutions for her in mainstream medicine. We knew we were buying time to find a better treatment, something beyond what was available in conventional medical practice that could address the *cause* of the disease rather than just suppress its manifestations by using toxic drugs that could kill her.

Synchronicity comes to Vicki's rescue

As fate would have it, shortly after this episode, one of my new patients requested that I interpret a test that another physician had ordered and that I'd never heard of. It was called the ELISA/ACT test.[1] Curious, I contacted the originating laboratory in Reston, Virginia, named Serammune Physicians Lab, and reached its medical director, Russell Jaffe, MD. Fortunately for us, he was planning to be in San Francisco in two weeks, and he offered to meet me in person while in town.

Russ disclosed the details about the test over a dinner at our home that lasted until midnight. He explained that his laboratory separates out the lymphocytes (a type of white blood cell in the immune system), which carry the memory of allergic reactions, and then incubates them in separate "wells" with one of 360 common substances to which many people have allergic reactions. Using this technique makes it simple to identify which wells display an immune reaction and thereby to discover the substances to which Vicki's immune system was reacting.

Could this be the test that Vicki needed to identify the elusive chemicals that were causing her anaphylactic reactions? After I shared Vicki's story with Russ, he immediately exclaimed, "Of course, and now you understand what this test is about!" The goal of the test was, he said, to "lower the antigenic load." In other words, his ELISA/ACT test first identified the chemicals (antigens) to which Vicki's immune system was reacting. The next step was to eliminate further exposure to them, thereby reducing the acute stimulus to her immune system. Simple common sense! He pointed out that if we *dealt with this underlying cause* rather than simply suppressing its symptoms with harmful drugs, we might eliminate her problem entirely.

Russ's test was unique—certainly far different from the extensive conventional skin and blood allergy testing that Vicki had undergone. Conventional tests at the time were limited to acute anaphylactic reactions caused by a specific class of antibody called IgE. However, Russ's test was designed to identify delayed anaphylactic reactions caused by a previously unknown immune mechanism.

Vicki's ELISA/ACT test soon determined that she had 41 allergies to common foods, skin care products, and many chemicals that are difficult to avoid in everyday life. Vicki was experiencing *delayed hypersensitivity reactions* to common chemicals that previous conventional tests had failed to identify because they were not measuring the right immune reaction. It is a good thing we discovered Russ and his cutting-edge test when we did, or Vicki might not be alive today.

But this was not all. Russ went on to explain that Vicki's delayed allergic responses were most likely caused by problems originating in her intestinal tract.

"Now you've gone too far—this sounds ridiculous!" I exclaimed. "I never learned this in my medical training. How could the intestinal tract have anything to do with anaphylaxis?"

"When chemicals to which we are sensitive enter the intestinal tract," he replied, "they can cause the development of abnormally large spaces between the cells that line the intestinal wall. This increases its permeability. An enormous influx of large molecules are then able to cross over and stimulate an immune response. Sometimes even whole bacteria have been documented to cross through these massively enlarged pores. One of the best-kept secrets in medicine is that the intestinal tract harbors about 60 percent of all the immune cells in the human body."

He explained further that, in this setting, the immune system can be dramatically overstimulated. It will mount an attack against these "alien" molecules and set the stage for a severe anaphylactic reaction. The coup de grace was that Vicki's test for intestinal permeability proved to be highly abnormal; she was indeed suffering from a severe form of *leaky gut syndrome*.[2]

We worked meticulously to eliminate Vicki's vulnerability to all her newly found chemical sensitivities over the next nine months. On the few occasions when we went to a restaurant, we brought a specially prepared meal from home that we could be certain did not have even a trace of the chemicals that were allergens for her. She read the ingredients in everything she purchased and learned to avoid all 41 substances to which she was allergic.

Now departing entirely from the regime that involved suppression of symptoms with synthetic chemicals, we also treated her with a specialized program of unusual nutritional supplements designed to stop ongoing allergic reactions that were injuring her intestinal tract. This program included probiotics (friendly bacteria that normally reside in the intestinal tract), L-glutamine (an amino acid), large doses of oral vitamin C, quercetin (a potent anti-inflammatory nutrient found in plants that also blocks allergic reactions), and Seacure (peptides from a white fish that support the repair of the damaged intestinal lining). Within a few weeks, Vicki was able to safely stop all of her pharmaceutical drugs, including the Prednisone that was causing so many serious problems. She has had no further anaphylactic attacks since that time, although she continues to use a few nutritional supplements to protect her intestinal tract and immune system. In short, she returned to a normal lifestyle, and her allergies have completely disappeared. It seemed like a miracle that Vicki fully recovered from what might have turned out to be a fatal disease if treated under the old medical paradigm.

Vicki's life was forever changed by this experience. It has in fact made her into a living example of a central message of this book: the imperative of taking personal responsibility for living a healthy lifestyle, along with the quest for *natural and nutritional solutions that address the cause of disease* instead of resorting to toxic drugs that only suppress symptoms. She now eats fresh, whole, organic food, uses organic personal skin care products that are biodegradable and nontoxic, and avoids exposure to environmental toxins as best as she can. We use a HEPA air purifier, rely on environmentally safe paints and carpets, and filter our home water supply. We even use a chlorine filter for baths and showers. Over the past 17 years, Vicki has compiled an extensive list of nontoxic cosmetics and household products that we've shared with innumerable people.

Dealing with the impact of our industrialized environment on our health is another essential component of the integral-health medicine model I present in this book, which seeks out causes coming from all possible domains. Vicki's near-death experience vividly taught me the importance of the issue of environmental toxins and the body's need for pure food and water. It also highlighted mainstream medicine's inability to deal effectively with the consequences of environmental toxicity in and around the body.[3]

A turning point in my relationship to medicine

The process of solving Vicki's life-threatening illness marked a major turning point in my medical career; my practice would never be the same. I knew that there was no going back. I had gone beyond my conventional training, tested new and uncharted waters, and begun an exploration in new fields of medicine that offered exciting possibilities. I could not turn away from what I had witnessed and what had likely saved my wife's life.

I soon immersed myself in learning more about natural and noninvasive ways to support and protect the body—taking courses, reading books and journals, and later searching the

Internet. By early 1994, I felt confident that what I had learned was safe, effective, and affordable. And I was convinced that it was a better style of medical practice than what I had learned in my formal medical training. Little did I know that this was just the beginning of my journey toward embracing a more expanded paradigm—one that aims to restore an optimal environment in the body by treating it with substances *natural* to the body.

Working up the strength to practice this new style of medicine was not easy—it took courage. Finally, I came out of the closet. I announced to my patients and colleagues that I would be incorporating lifestyle management and natural therapies before resorting to the more aggressive style I'd been taught in my training, the allopathic approach that depends so heavily on drugs, technologies, and surgeries.

At the same time, however, I was fearful that my peers and patients would think I'd gone off the deep end. I imagined that my medical partners would ask me to leave our group practice, that I might lose my medical license for practicing unconventional medicine, and that my patients might abandon me. Not much of that happened, at least not at the start. In fact, in the beginning, both my patients and colleagues were intrigued by my new, more eclectic approach and encouraged me to continue. But that sentiment would prove to be short-lived.

Throughout this period of expansive growth, I continued to appreciate the value of conventional medicine. My mission at first was a quest to integrate the best from conventional medicine with the best from the new natural medicine as well as other forms of CAM (complementary and alternative medicine), and to carefully blend these styles of practice to support the needs of my patients. I was beginning to embrace integrative medicine as the new model. And I was soon to develop an even more advanced model of care that I now call integral-health medicine.

I learn a key premise
of the new medical paradigm

Russ Jaffe had introduced me to a new model of the practice of medicine, and he was well qualified to do it. He had received his MD degree from the Boston University School of Medicine in 1972 and completed his residency training in clinical pathology at the National Institutes of Health, where he was on the permanent staff as a practicing molecular biologist and molecular pathologist. In addition, he had studied nutrition extensively. In 1978, Russ was invited to become the founding chairman of the Scientific Committee of the American Holistic Medical Association by Norm Shealy, MD, its cofounder.

In the 1970s, Russ had also joined another group of pioneers known as the Society for Orthomolecular Health Medicine (OHM Society).[3] This group focused on going beyond treating patients with drugs and technologies that in general suppress symptoms of disease, and began investigating how to deal with their underlying causes. Led by two-time Nobel Prize winner Linus Pauling, the OHM Society looked primarily to natural, rather than synthetic, molecules to support the restoration and maintenance of good health. Today the group is led by one of my closest friends and mentors, Richard Kunin, MD.

This style of natural medicine focuses on factors that influence cell biochemistry and searches for *natural* biochemical solutions that support the body's innate ability to restore normal cellular biochemistry and healthy physiology. Orthomolecular physicians operate from the premise that if all the body's cells are functioning perfectly, it is impossible to be sick. Surprisingly, there are only a few ways that a cell's normal function can be disturbed, as we will see later. The restoration of good health and vitality is accomplished by supporting the body and allowing the natural healing process to take charge. Realizing this principle was crucial in opening my eyes to the emerging new paradigm of healing and medicine.

Nature has always done the healing

I now know that it is entirely wrongheaded to discount the importance of the natural healing abilities that operate so miraculously within each of us. It makes sense to manage our colds by eliminating their symptoms, but it also makes far more sense to address the underlying issue that led to the weakening of our natural immunity. We all know that lifestyle factors such as diet, sleep, exercise, and stress have important roles in regulating our immunity. Even so, the disease care model of medicine barely gives lip service to these commonsense lifestyle practices.

Even though substantial data supports the value and safety of natural medicine remedies and other alternative modalities, and decades of research prove the centrality of lifestyle factors in maintaining health and supporting immunity, such things are simply not what physicians are trained to prescribe or promote. It hardly seems fair, after all they've gone through to become physicians, to ask them to return to school to learn a whole new medical paradigm. But providing good medicine is not about being fair to physicians—nor is it about assigning fault. It is about doing what is right and best for our patients.

And what is best for our patients, as I was to learn from our Health Medicine Forums and from my own research and decades of clinical experience, is a model for health care based on the four basic principles of integral-health medicine—care that is *integrative, holistic, person-centered*, and *preventive*. These concepts are explored in detail later in the book.

Furthermore, true healing is a process that also includes our exploration of the *meaning* of illness. This dimension *includes but transcends* the physical and emotional domains of any illness, and is integrally involved with our whole life story, as well as our relationship to our environment, society, and culture—even our relationship to everything that exists in the cosmos.

As I review my own situation, I'm amazed that I was somehow able to step out of the conventional medical box to reassess how I was practicing medicine and go beyond my training to embrace a new paradigm. No doubt, my wife's illness was a major catalyst. But there were others, such as learning how to stretch beyond my limitations as a tennis athlete, and my underlying dissatisfaction with medicine, dating back to medical school (which I chronicle in chapter 2). Few practicing physicians have made this transition from disease care to genuine health care, and even fewer have been successful at it. For the most part, I had to undergo this transformation without the support of my colleagues or my profession. Even today, more than 15 years later, few physicians are willing to practice the new medicine or are even willing to collaborate with practitioners who do. But I hope and believe that this reluctance will soon give way to the inevitable.

Resistance against the new medicine

Allow me to emphasize again: Despite its clinical successes and its increasing scientific validation worldwide, there continues to be serious resistance on the part of the mainstream to bringing the new medicine—in its various forms and models—forward into clinical practice. It has been especially difficult to introduce it into our hospitals, as I explain later.

While there is nothing intrinsically wrong with managing symptoms of disease, this practice by itself is a dangerously limited approach. As the great Albert Schweitzer once stated, "It's supposed to be a secret, but I'll tell you anyway. We doctors do nothing. We only help and encourage the doctor within." Of course, Schweitzer was referring to the innate ability of the body to restore and maintain its own good health when given the opportunity and the proper support.

Conventional medicine focuses instead almost exclusively on managing symptoms. And it does this for a reason: Scientific research has been unable to discover the root causes for most diseases. But deep economic, political, and cultural factors also account for mainstream medicine's glaring omission of support for the body's ability to self-heal.

Sadly, not only are mainstream physicians *not* trained in techniques for strengthening the body's defenses, but also they receive no training in detoxification—nearly a foreign word in conventional medical training. It is amazing that the role of toxins in our body in creating disease, and the importance of eliminating them or external sources of toxins (as in the case of Vicki), is for the most part completely overlooked in medical training. Perhaps this should not be so surprising, since the role of nutrition is also largely ignored as well.

Nonetheless, treating symptoms has its benefits. Helping people to feel better is not a bad thing! We all want to feel well, especially when we are sick. If there is a way to make us feel better in the short term, who would turn it down? It is for this very reason that medical research based in the disease care paradigm has been so avidly supported by the American public. Never before in our history have we had such a powerful armamentarium of drugs and technologies to help us *feel better.*

Of course, the problem with this approach is that we've gone far overboard. We've failed to recognize that our symptoms are indispensable guides to those issues or behaviors in our lives that require our full attention. They often point to deep inner places where healing needs to occur or where we must make improvements in our lifestyle practices, our social and cultural systems, or our larger physical environment.

Thus, in our single-minded search for shortcuts to relief, we are missing the lessons our symptoms seek to provide for us, and we are compounding our problems in our ignorance. Americans have even turned in droves to antidepressants and antianxiety drugs to suppress our psychospiritual problems, even though such concerns belong in the domain of psychology, religion, and spirituality; a disturbing part of this trend is that psychiatrists have almost entirely shifted their emphasis from psychotherapy to psychopharmacology—even those who work with children!

It is both sad and remarkable that we have been content to turn to drugs that suppress our symptoms—or give the illusion of doing so—and we take so little responsibility for measures that are simple and commonsense ways of keeping ourselves healthy and our society highly functioning. And that leaves aside the consideration that such drugs can be inordinately expensive, add toxicity to the body, and come with a risk of serious and even life-threatening side effects, as we explore in chapter 5.

Getting back to the basics of health

A first step is to get back to basics—back to nature herself. Humankind has evolved in a complicated, symbiotic, and dynamic relationship with nature over thousands of years. We have adapted to what nature has provided for us in the way of food, herbs, water, air, and everything else that exists on our planet. Over the millennia, we have successfully made genetic changes that have allowed us to live in harmony with our natural environment. No wonder indigenous healers believe that for every human illness there is an herbal remedy. Even today, the vast majority of our most powerful pharmaceutical drugs are derived from plants and herbs.

But because of commercial pressure and cultural prejudice, many Americans ignore the value of natural foods and herbs in supporting wellness and treating disease. Far too many of us, including physicians, have forgotten what Hippocrates said 2,500 years ago: "Let food be thy medicine and medicine be thy food." While high-quality food and herbs may not solve all health care problems, they are certainly the right place to start. It would be a giant step forward if our hospitals, for example, were to follow Hippocrates' advice and begin treatment of all patients with a healthy diet that is oriented to their special nutritional needs. It makes one wonder what is going on in the minds of our hospital staffs that provide sick patients with fast foods that are low in nutrients and fiber, and high in calories, pesticides, insecticides, fungicides, preservatives, and even trans fats and high-fructose corn sugar!

Even if we have failed to maintain a healthy lifestyle, there is almost always hope for natural means of improvement in our health. Our bodies can adapt physically in remarkable ways if we give them a chance. If we exercise our bodies, they respond by increasing their reserve capacity in dramatic ways, as I explain in chapter 6. We can substantially increase the reserves and strength of our cardiac, pulmonary, muscular, mental, visual, and so many other systems simply by working out regularly. The old adage "Use it or lose it" is precisely true. Even people with congestive heart failure can use exercise to lessen the severity of their problem. Our physical bodies are fantastic in their ability to adapt to the demands of sensible, regular exercise.

As we age, it is absolutely critical that we get the most out of our bodies by continuing to exercise. It is remarkable what an older athlete can do compared with younger people who are couch potatoes—I know from experience. We have extensive data showing that even minimal exercise will extend life and reduce morbidity to a remarkable degree. And the more vigorous the exercise, the better we condition ourselves. Not everyone needs to be a competitive athlete, but those who exercise well and do more of it will generally be stronger and healthier and enjoy a much longer and higher-quality life.

Getting enough sleep and reducing stress are also basic commonsense strategies that make us feel better, allow us to stay healthier, and extend our life span. We've known for a long time that adequate sleep is essential to health and longevity. For example, the American Cancer Society conducted a study in the 1950s on more than a million people that considered the effects of exercise, nutrition, smoking, and sleep on health. It found that over a seven-year period, those people who got less than four hours a night of sleep had the highest mortality rates among all these factors. Lack of sleep suppresses our immunity and increases our risk for diabetes, osteoporosis, hypertension, obesity, heart attacks, strokes, and many other diseases.

Along with observing the prerequisite of healthy lifestyle practices, it is also time for Americans to go back to the basics of using simple, noninvasive, and safe health care strategies before resorting to potentially dangerous drugs, technologies, and surgeries. We have been seduced into depending almost exclusively on these invasive modalities rather than on time-tested natural approaches, many of which have been passed down from generation to generation for thousands of years, and which are concerned with bringing the whole person back into balance. These approaches include acupuncture, homeopathy, nutrition, energy medicine, chiropractic, bodywork, imagery, biofeedback, hypnotherapy, aromatherapy, and so much more.

We must treat the whole person

Human beings are an *inseparable* combination of body, mind, emotion, and spirit, as these are embedded in society, culture, and the universe. That's the way we are hard-wired. Every person is unique with respect to who she is in each of these special domains. And we all deserve nothing less than to be treated from the standpoint of all these perspectives. Each of the aspects of who and what we are provides a window through which we can be observed and assessed by our physicians and, ultimately, by ourselves. The more information our physicians collect from each of these perspectives, the greater the opportunity to create strategies to support the return to optimal health. It is also the responsibility of the physician to partner with us in order to understand our health issues and cocreate the best solutions.

One day, a radical reform of health care will provide us all with such an approach.

And now, let's step back a moment for a look at my own lengthy journey—first away from, and then back toward, these very insights.

Two

How I Became Part of the Problem: The Story of My Medical Training

*The crucial ingredient of an integral medical practice
is not the integral medical bag itself—but the holder of that bag.*

—Ken Wilber, from the foreword to *Consciousness and Healing*

Some babies are born with their umbilical cord wrapped around their neck. I must have come in with stethoscope tubing around mine. I was probably destined to learn that medicine can offer us a nourishing lifeline—or it might just as easily coil around our necks and choke the life out of us!

The story of my training and subsequent four decades of medical practice provides testimony that modern medicine has indeed become a source of great hope *and* great danger.

In this chapter, we will start by examining the ironies involved in my "unhealthy" medical training during the 1960s. This training regime, which was marked by intimidation and even outright abusive practices and the inculcation of unhealthy attitudes toward ourselves and our patients, culminated in my effort in

1970 to unionize local interns and residents at a hospital where I was chief resident. Our challenge to a virtually misanthropic system became part of a short-lived but dramatic nationwide effort to change the nature of medical training and practice. We ultimately failed, but we set a historic precedent that is a valuable lesson in today's struggle for radical health care reform.

Len will grow up to be a doctor!

As far back as I can remember—even before kindergarten—everyone in my family took it as a fact of life that "when Len grows up, he will be a physician." Yet something deep inside me resisted, even held me back through medical school. I knew I was *supposed* to become a successful doctor, but I didn't *want* to be one—I wanted to be a professional tennis player!

Even as a child, I enjoyed sports more than school. I was good at most of them because I was agile and quick. After school I'd stay until just before dinner, playing almost any kind of sport. Even my summers were spent playing baseball, basketball, or football. But it wasn't until I was 16 that I had the opportunity to learn how to play tennis. When I finally did, I knew right away that tennis would be my sport. In fact, within just two weeks of taking up tennis, I was ready to try out for my high school team. I played number two singles that year; and the next year, my senior year, I won the county singles championship, though I lost badly in the regionals.

I made the freshman tennis team when I entered the University of California, Berkeley, but did not earn my varsity letter until my senior year, when we finished third in the NCAA tournament. However, that was it for tennis for the time being; I was now off to medical school. For the next ten years, I hardly picked up a racket more than once a month, but I never lost interest in the game.

When I completed my medical training in internal medicine in 1971, I opened a practice in Walnut Creek, California, at John Muir Medical Center. I had married while in med school, and by now I had two young children. But having finished my years of medical training and residency finally left me a little free time. It was time to return to tennis! It wasn't long before I was playing most days after work and began feeling the itch to compete.

Somehow, in the midst of starting up my medical practice and returning to tennis, I became sidetracked with an even more ambitious idea: building my own tennis club. Not just any tennis club, but one with 37 tennis courts, 13 of which were indoors; one indoor court that could seat 5,000 people and host Davis Cup matches; plus 30,000 square feet of clubhouse that had all kinds of social and other amenities. By 1973, my two business partners and I had a building permit for a $5.5 million facility and most of the financing to build it. But as luck would have it, interest rates suddenly went from 8 to 18 percent just before the deal was finalized, stopping us in our tracks. Plans for the club were shifted to a modest outdoor facility that today is just another tennis club in Walnut Creek. Nonetheless, I was back playing competitive tennis by the time this ordeal was over.

Are you wondering how I could do all this and still have time for a wife and children? Had I turned into a machine that was on automatic pilot to achieve goals rather than be with the most important people in my life? Was I out of control in terms of having balance in my life? And is it any wonder that in 1976 my then-wife asked for a divorce?

A decade passed before I fully understood what had happened, allowing me to renew my search for a more meaningful purpose in life.

The years continued to pass, and I married again. By the end of the first 25 years of my medical career, I had become a highly respected doctor *and* was ranked number one in the world in competitive senior tennis. But what had I really accomplished? Was the world a big tennis court? Was a successful medical practice truly something that was measured by mastery of the technology to treat diseases and by the respect of my peers?

It was 1990 before I began shifting my interest from the practice of tennis to medicine and the way *it* was practiced. While I continued playing tournament tennis—in fact, some of my best tennis ever—I was also beginning to see the need for radical change in our health care system and even the paradigm of medicine itself. Tennis had taught me that it takes far more than skill to excel; it also takes enormous passion, heart, and self-confidence. My fierce determination to excel in tennis now somehow carried over to my practice of medicine and then to the discovery of my life purpose of *improving the way that medicine is practiced.*

This purpose, arriving late in my life, must have been the unconscious reason why I had initially chosen the path to medicine, but it was not apparent until several decades into my medical career. The truth is, I didn't enjoy my medical training or even the early years of my practice. Deep down I knew during those years that there was something fundamentally wrong with our health care system. I was not ready to act on what I saw, but those early experiences served as a baseline from which I would one day compare how medicine is practiced with how it must be transformed.

Isn't it strange how our lives unfold in a way that allows us to discover our true inner selves? For me, it was necessary to first become a world champion tennis player; this allowed me to prove to myself that I could do whatever I wanted in life. No, it wouldn't simply be because "Len was supposed to become a doctor" that he actually *was* one!

Finally, the stethoscope tubing around my neck had loosened, and I was reborn, free to choose my own destiny—that of recovering the soul of medicine and radically reforming our health care system.

True medicine is about healing—isn't it?

Today my bottom line is simple: *Medicine should be about healing.* It's about caring for the ordinary people who come to us seeking care and enjoying the process of helping them to become whole again.

The physician-healer should be deeply interested in knowing why patients hold certain beliefs and how what they believe leads them to make choices that affect their total health. Further, to be able to heal, we as healers need to walk in our patients' shoes. Seeing the world through their eyes is essential if we are to truly know our patients, discover what they want, and find out just how to help them achieve physical, mental, emotional, and spiritual health as contributing members of a healthy community.

When I was a young man entering medical training, my idealistic image of a physician had always been of an understanding, giving, and wise human being. Physicians might work long hours and were sometimes sleep-deprived, I thought, yet they were always there to treat and comfort those in need. I wanted to be like that someday. I wanted to help people live happy, healthy, meaningful lives. I was definitely intrigued by the high-tech nature of the science of medicine, but I also had a deep and genuine interest in doing more than just fixing people's symptoms. I wanted to be a healer, but medical training directly subverted this natural desire.

Medical school may be hazardous to your health

When I entered Duke University Medical School, I fully expected my graduate and postgraduate training to be challenging. I was excited because finally, after waiting my whole life, I'd be entering into the brotherhood of physicians—a community of healers. I discovered to my shock that the educational regime's central aim, in effect, was to create a "community" of alienated, inauthentic, and unhealed "scientists."

The few professors who were patient and empathetic inspired us students to work even harder. But inspiration was rarely the motivating factor in our training. Too often we were driven by fear—in particular, fear of humiliation. When we made errors because of a lack of knowledge or experience, we were often ridiculed in front of our colleagues and patients. This practice encouraged us to hide our lack of knowledge for fear of being embarrassed.

Does this account sound overstated or perhaps out of date? Consider some current data from a study of 2,884 medical students from 16 nationally representative U.S. medical schools from the class of 2003 that was published in the *British Medical Journal* in September 2006. The authors of the study concluded, "Most medical students in the United States report having been harassed or belittled during their training. Although few students characterized the harassment or belittlement as severe, poor mental health and low career satisfaction were significantly correlated with these experiences."

There's more. An October 2008 *New York Times* article on medical student burnout reported:

> In 2006, Dr. Liselotte N. Dyrbye and her colleagues at the Mayo Clinic found that nearly half of the 545 medical students they surveyed suffered from burnout, which they defined as professional distress in three domains: emotional exhaustion, depersonalization, and low sense of personal accomplishment. Moreover, the researchers found that each successive year of schooling increased the chances students would experience burnout, despite the fact that they had entered medical school with mental health profiles similar to those of their peers who chose other career paths.
>
> More recently . . . Dr. Dyrbye and her colleagues widened the scope of their research, analyzing survey responses from 2,248 medical students at seven medical schools across the country. Again, nearly half of the students surveyed met the criteria for burnout. But the investigators discovered an even

more ominous finding: 11 percent of all the students surveyed also reported having suicidal thoughts in the past year. . . .

In a third study, Dr. Dyrbye found that when tested for empathy, medical students at baseline generally scored higher than their nonmedical peers. But, as medical students experienced more burnout, *there was a corresponding drop in the level of empathy toward patients* [emphasis added].[2]

If this is the result of medical training even today, what sort of premise must underline this approach? And how entrenched is it?

Suffice it to say for now that it is impossible for physicians to do a good job of guiding patients through tough health care challenges when they have little confidence in what they know, have emotional scars from their training, and may have fallen out of touch with their own inner growth as individuals.

Ironically, training of this kind may lead physicians to give the impression that they know everything when they don't. Perhaps this explains why some physicians act defensively and arrogantly when questioned about a given treatment plan they have recommended. The record shows that such attitudes lead to misrepresentations, treatment failures, disappointment, anger, and lawsuits.

Being a clinician is about becoming increasingly human

Let's delve into this a little more deeply. Living as an ordinary human being means, at least in part, accepting human limitations. No doctor, not even a board-certified specialist, can expect to be omniscient in his or her field; we are all limited, erring, and finite beings. And no one today can master more than a minuscule percentage of the entire medical literature—there is just too much of it. Studies have documented that unless physicians read in the vicinity of 50 medical articles a day in just their pertise, they fall behind the cutting edge. Of course, ly are not enough hours in the day for anyone to do also practicing medicine. But what we *can* realistically provide our patients beyond our knowledge or training, which is necessarily incomplete, is our *entire being*—our full attention and our full humanity.

How does this apply to medical training? Mastering the information in textbooks and journals is difficult, but applying our limited knowledge to clinical situations is an even greater challenge. And while a certain amount of scientific and technical knowledge is essential to practicing good medicine, I've come to realize that it is far more important that medical students learn about *being human*. This surely means that, in their training, they must be given the space and encouragement to grow into healthy, balanced people—and hopefully walk a spiritual path of their choosing. Otherwise, how can they grow to be physician-healers? Some measure of wisdom and emotional maturity is essential if a doctor is going to be able to provide patients with guidance around health and healing. Really helping patients—at least as primary care providers—requires that our input be not only well thought out and informed by the latest science, but also steeped in the lessons of our own life experiences.

If facts and techniques were all that were necessary to solve medical problems, computers would be all we'd need to treat sick people. Of course, this is simply not the case, and until we have computers that emulate a physician who can feel deeply and use judgment based on personal experience and reflection, no software program will ever be able to practice good medicine.

This gets us to the bottom line: In medicine, the central issue we face is the utter uniqueness of each individual person amid the dynamic nature of his health challenges in the moment—and all this is best seen within the larger context of his specific family commitments, social roles, and cultural predispositions. This inherent condition of clinical practice guarantees that the same set of facts often does not lead to the same treatment plan. And that's why we as physician-healers *have to be fully present with our patients.* We must offer ourselves as we actually are in the moment, be clear about our abilities and limitations, and create a level playing field with our patients. In the doctor–patient relationship, healing is a process that can occur only in a sacred space shared by two authentic human beings; neither is superior, and both are committed to understanding and supporting one another as they explore options for transforming illness into optimal health.

Humility is a central quality of excellence in medicine

Being authentic should be highly valued, encouraged, and respected in all areas of life, not just in the medical field. As Socrates pointed out long ago, knowing that we *do not know*—and being clear about it—is not a weakness; it's a virtue, a sign of strength of character. It's an indicator of an inner commitment to finding the truth. Giving a false impression that we know something when we don't, or that we are something that we aren't, is a sign of weakness of character.

The authenticity that arises from true humility is essential, of course, when it involves medical treatment that may make the difference between living or dying.

How can we as physicians incorporate clear boundaries between what we do and do not know, and what we are and are not, and still have confidence that we can practice high-quality medicine? Every medical school faculty member should be teaching and modeling authentic behavior at all times. We are all human beings, whether patients or students, and we deserve nothing less than the right to tell the truth without fear of punishment. It is not realistic to expect young physicians in training to learn how to become healers if they are programmed to operate from fear of failure rather than the virtue of humility and the desire to simply be of service.

I have often wondered if it is partly due to this training in ingrained fear and alienation that today's physicians have failed to stick together and stand up against the ravages of managed care medicine. It may also be a contributing factor to why physicians have such a high incidence of failed marriages, substance abuse, depression, and suicide.

Put another way, if we want physicians who are understanding and compassionate, it is critical that we train our medical students with the same respect and compassion that we aim to provide for our patients. We cannot expect our physicians to model or teach patients what they do not know from personal experience and training. It is even more difficult for physicians to guide patients in the ultimate journey of healing and personal growth if they are not on an authentic journey of their own.

A startling case of my own depersonalization in medical training

Looking back, it is clear that my own training worked in the opposite direction. For example, as medical students, we were sometimes required to do experiments on ourselves that showed little respect for our value as human beings. In one instance, our entire class was required to ingest sulfonamide antibiotic tablets and then measure our urinary excretion rate over the next several hours. This was in theory a valuable teaching experience—as we'd surely remember an experiment we did on ourselves—but there were worrisome safety issues.

I requested to be excused from this experiment; I knew that at least 10 percent of our class would be at risk of developing a significant allergic or toxic reaction from the medication. However, if we wanted to get credit for this class, we had to take the sulfa pills and complete the experiment. Reluctantly, I took the pills. I hadn't gotten this far in my training just to quit because of one experiment!

As fate would have it, within three minutes of ingesting the pills, I broke out in hives and was itching all over. I immediately reported this to my professor, who sent me to student health by myself to get some antihistamine pills. I took a pill and returned in less than five minutes, during which the rash had spread from my head to my toes. Suddenly I began to feel that I was moving in slow motion. I became weak and lightheaded, vomited, and lost consciousness.

When the seriousness of the anaphylactic reaction I was having was appreciated, I was rushed to the intensive care unit. I was immediately given intravenous fluids, oxygen, and more antiallergic medications, and was observed for a few hours. Later that day, I was discharged home and advised to take a few more antihistamines over the next day or two. I had no further follow-up or treatment and was never asked how I was doing after that time. No follow-up laboratory work was performed, as normally should be done. It was simply assumed that I'd be fine. I did recover fully, but it certainly felt like no one cared about me as person.

This deplorable incident had an upside. The class learned that it's dangerous to put synthetic chemicals in our bodies, and we should not minimize unnecessary risks when giving them to patients. This was a lesson I learned repeatedly as a practicing physician, and it had a powerful but delayed impact on how I would practice medicine decades later. Every time a physician prescribes a medication for a patient, an experiment is being undertaken. No two people are alike, and there is no way to know in advance with absolute certainty whether or not a serious or even life-threatening side effect will occur.

Within two years of this incident, the pharmacology curriculum no longer included measuring urinary excretion rates following ingestion of sulfonamide antibiotics. I'd like to think it was because the teaching staff was primarily concerned about our welfare rather than medical legal consequences they might have faced if someone had been seriously injured or even died from this unnecessary and dangerous experiment.

I've often wondered what could have been going on in our professors' minds. They obviously were interested in teaching us about pharmacokinetics, but where was the concern for our personal welfare? When we became medical students, had we stopped being looked upon as human beings? Had we become mere instruments for teaching? Was our training to be like a series of sadistic episodes out of the TV series *Scrubs*? You would hope that medical training for a precious new generation of healers would highlight appreciation of the value of human life and human comfort.

Learning how to become a healer begins with learning to value and respect one's own self first! We'll examine more about what makes a true healer in later chapters.

More depersonalization
in working with live patients

Of course, our misanthropic medical training did not stop there. During the last two years of medical school, we were introduced to clinical training and began working with patients on the hospital wards. No more classes with cadavers, no more experiments on animals, and no more risky experiments on ourselves. We were actually going to learn from living people with real diseases.

At our hospital, patients were grouped together in large wards with 15 or more patients in long rows of beds adjacent to one another. A cloth curtain could be drawn around each bed that would allow some degree of privacy. Behind a drawn curtain, somewhere between three and ten teachers and students would often gather around the crowded bedside to review each patient's health problems. Our professors would ask patients a few pertinent questions, examine them in front of the entire group to demonstrate the key features of each person's disease, and ask us questions about the particular disease in question and how we'd approach managing it.

To my surprise, we engaged in "scientific" discussions about the diseases these unfortunate and very sick patients had, often as though they were not even there. They were just invisible "cases"— not the concerned, sick individuals that peered into our eyes, searching for hope and compassion. While the patients were all treated politely, they were not treated personally or respectfully. We were being trained to become *detached* from our patients. We were learning to treat diseases rather than human beings; we were in fact learning to be *scientists*, not healers, who were operating according to the protocols and premises of the disease care system.

None of us dared to question this "wisdom," but I remember wondering: How could we be healers if we didn't even know our patients as real people? How could our patients have trust in us if they didn't know us, or we them? Yet in my mind I can still hear the echoes of our professors repeatedly warning: "Be scientific and objective. Stay detached from your patients. Do not get personally involved in their lives. You must remain objective to be a scientist, and physicians above all must be scientists."

Now, more than 40 years later, I see how deeply misguided this concept of training was. As an experienced clinician, I find it difficult to even *imagine* practicing medicine without developing meaningful personal relationships with my patients. Allow me to repeat: Healing relationships develop from a dialogue built upon mutual trust; from a willingness to be authentic and vulnerable; and from sharing information, attitudes, and feelings with each other as equals. Each patient is unique and has special personal needs. Developing a healing relationship requires creating a sacred space that allows a connection at a deep personal level and a willingness to work together to find the best solution. Healing is a collaborative, deliberative process that engages patient and healer at the deepest levels of human existence.

The theme of separation
is at the heart of the medical model

Throughout my training at Duke Medical School, the dualism of separation was incessantly programmed into our minds. In fact, it became a central theme. We were taught separation from each other, separation from our patients, separation from our instructors, separation of mind from body, and separation from all disciplines that did not stem from so-called evidenced-based mainstream medicine. Indeed, we were being trained in the fundamental attitude of the practice of modern medicine itself: separation from *nature*. We were taught to be at war with disease, and proclaimed ourselves to be the only profession competent to carry the flag and fight the battle against disease.

Medicine was to be a separated and detached genre, and we were being prepared to enter the impersonal, lonely, and sterile world of "the scientific method." What we could not either dissect or test in the laboratory, or conceptually understand using our Newtonian, reductionistic approach, was simply ignored or thrown out of the medical domain and dismissed as neither relevant nor important.

We were also learning to operate as if in a vacuum, isolated from all other health care practices and professions. We were taught to have great pride in being physicians, as we were repeatedly reminded that we were "the best trained of all health care professionals."

In fact, all other forms of health care practice were regarded as subordinate to the practice of medicine. When they supposedly defied scientific analysis, they were for the most part categorically dismissed. They were assumed to be not just valueless, but a sham or possibly even harmful.

We were brainwashed into believing that chiropractors were unscrupulous quacks who treated diseases such as cancer by manipulation of the spine and who were duping innocent fools into believing that their "dangerous" manipulations did something worthwhile. We were taught that homeopathy couldn't possibly have a scientific effect because drugs are not used in most homeopathic remedies, so how could they possibly have a biochemical effect on human physiology? Herbal medicine was for savages who did not have the sophistication to refine herbs to make pharmaceutical drugs. Acupuncture was not scientifically tested, so why should we even consider it? Indeed, no alternative discipline was regarded as offering anything of much value. Today, of course, we know that few attitudes are more outrageous and unscientific than this kind of professional arrogance.

When I asked my professors about how some of these disciplines worked, to my surprise they did not seem to know much. I found that they knew little beyond the boundaries of their own limited medical training. I wondered how they could be so certain that these disciplines, some of which had been around for millennia, were useless or even dangerous. In those days, I did not have the courage to pursue this line of questioning. Why aggravate the people who would be giving me grades and were already making life difficult enough for me?

Preparing to be a research scientist at the NIH

Even more mistreatment was to befall me in my training. At one point in my education at Duke Medical School, I contemplated becoming a research scientist. In my third year, I entered Duke's prestigious Research Training Program and prepared for a scientific career with the National Institutes of Health (NIH), as did many top students at Duke. Toward that end, in July 1965 I began a highly coveted internship at a medical center that shall remain nameless. Within two weeks after I started this program, my wife announced that she had had enough of life with a two-year-old and a husband who was never home. She was going to return to California and wanted to know if I was going to join her and our son.

I thought it best to share this news with the chief of the department of medicine, hoping that he'd somehow help me resolve this situation. And what a disaster that turned out to be! I still remember his words of advice: "Saputo, you have a bit of promise, but I'll assure you of one thing. If you leave this program, I'll see to it that you'll never pass your boards in internal medicine!" And at the time, he was the chairman of the National Board of Medical Examiners.

I was looking for compassion, support, fatherly advice. What I got was just the opposite. Nothing was more important to this pathetic "chief of medicine" than his precious training program. Actually, his lack of compassion made it easy to decide to leave and look for another internship in the San Francisco Bay Area. Within the next couple of days, I had secured an internship that was just a few miles from where my wife and I had grown up. It certainly was not the internship I'd hoped for, but it was close to both of our families, and it was available. It was not easy to give up an internship in internal medicine that almost certainly would have led to a promising career in research at the NIH and to instead enter into an internship at the county hospital in Oakland, California. Highland General Hospital (HGH) was about the last place anyone interested in becoming a research fellow at the NIH would consider attending. Remarkably, this turned out to be one of the best decisions of my life, because it redirected my training to the practice of medicine rather than the sterile world of medical research.

Severe sleep deprivation and medical postgraduate training

The experience of internship and residency training is a powerful way to learn medicine, but the sleep deprivation of interns and residents that goes with it is yet another indication of a medical system that harbors sadistic and unhealthy values. At HGH, we were put into the trenches of the hospital wards, where as young physicians we learned through intense experience how to manage a wide range of common and uncommon health conditions. But this education came at a high price—not just for us but for our patients as well—because HGH observed that crazy tradition according to which interns and residents must work up to 120-hour weeks for prolonged stretches. Our schedule often translated into being on call for 36 hours and then getting 12 hours off.

This practice is still engaged in nationwide, albeit in modified form. And the interns and residents are still paying a high price. In a Harvard study reported at the 21st Annual Meeting of the Associated Professional Sleep Societies in June 2007, the effects of insufficient sleep on 2,737 medical interns were studied.[3] When these young physicians worked five or more extended-duration shifts in a month, they reported seven times greater chances of making at least one medical error that resulted in an adverse patient event. They also reported a 300 percent increase in fatigue-related preventable adverse events that resulted in the death of a patient.

When I was in training, we all understood the unspoken code of "ethics" requiring that you never complain about personal sacrifice, even if it had the potential to compromise patient care. If we dared to take a stand against this policy, we knew that we'd be dismissed from the training program. Everyone knew that this tradition was dangerous and inappropriate, but we didn't have the courage to stand up against our teachers. Once again, we were operating from fear.

I certainly wouldn't have wanted to face my attending physician the next morning had I declined to admit a patient in the middle of the night because I was "too tired." I could just imagine hearing her saying, "Aren't you interested in your patients, doctor? Maybe you're not cut out to be a physician." I sometimes felt as if I were going through fraternity hell week, except that for interns and residents it wasn't just a week—we were browbeaten with this treatment for months on end.

When I think of some of the decisions we made during those challenging times, it's a miracle that so many of our patients survived! It was difficult enough to make the correct decisions when we were fresh and alert, let alone provide acute care in a state of chronic sleep deprivation.

In one very unusual situation during my residency, nature and sanity temporarily reasserted themselves, and I did get enough sleep. As a senior resident in internal medicine, I was assigned a short rotation at the local Veterans Administration hospital, where I was responsible for providing weekend medical coverage for the emergency room. On this particular weekend, I found an opportunity to take a short nap around 5 p.m. on a Saturday afternoon. We had rooms where we could catch up on sleep if the opportunity arose. This room had no windows and was totally blacked out, and I was exhausted. It took only a few seconds before I fell into a deep sleep.

When I was finally awakened, I was shocked to find out that it was Monday morning. I had slept for 38 straight hours! For reasons that I'll never understand, not a single patient who needed my services had come to the emergency room during this entire period. It was as though my guardian angel had said, "Enough! This is unfair. I'll make sure you get some sleep." Actually, I felt guilty for "sleeping on the job." But perhaps the universe had intervened to take care of me, and my patients too.

Looking back at this now, I can appreciate the value of getting used to the sometimes long and unpredictable hours that we faced in clinical practice; nevertheless, I consider this style of training abusive, unnecessary, and inappropriate. In the decades since my own training, these policies have changed somewhat. It is now against the rules of any medical teaching institution to require physicians in training to work more than 80 hours a week. Yet there are still reports of instances in training programs where much longer hours are required. I find it disheartening that some senior physicians and hospital administrators continue to take advantage of interns and residents rather than support them. This tradition persists for two major reasons: First, as is the case in families, abusive practices are easily handed down from generation to generation; and second, interns and residents are cheap labor. Far from being trained as healers, we were being exploited like sweatshop workers!

While it is common knowledge that teaching hospitals save a lot of money by using physicians in training to provide many patient services, it wasn't until April 2007 that an article was published in *Archives of Surgery* documenting the actual dollar amounts saved.[4] They determined that if surgical residents continued to work their usual 80-hour weeks but had 20 of those hours replaced by instruction rather than caring for patients—and if nurse practitioners were used to make up those 20 hours—over five years it would cost the hospitals an additional $1.9 million per resident. It doesn't take much to imagine the financial advantage of having a resident house staff of 100 people on any teaching hospital's budget.

Learning how to heal
through inspiration, not intimidation

The best way to teach healing is through inspiration and compassion, not intimidation, mistreatment, or unreasonable working conditions. A good medical education involves far more than learning medical facts and treatment techniques, and "working hard." Becoming a physician and a healer entails learning what life itself is about—including the nature of human consciousness and the role of spirituality in healing. It should include a search for the true nature of peak health and well-being, and a quest to find out what people need as whole beings. As I have pointed out, we can best learn these things by working to achieve balance in our own lives. Physicians in training, like everyone else, should have time for family life, exercise, meditation, and reflection, and at least a little allowance for recreation and relaxation.

It is both surprising and disappointing that older physicians who have gone through the rigors of medical training themselves and have been in practice for years have not taken action to ensure that every physician in training has a reasonably balanced life and is personally engaged in a journey of uncovering the secrets of longevity and wellness. Imagine what kind of health care system we would have if medical school professors came to the realization that teaching programs should be inspirational and should enhance the students' personal growth toward wholeness—with the goal of creating genuine healers!

The fact of the matter is that key concepts in healing—such as the nature of true wellness, peak health, and wholeness—cannot be taught solely from a book. These qualities of living must also be experienced. It is very difficult to teach what we do not understand from experience; we simply cannot give what we do not have. It should therefore not come as a surprise that physicians who lived an unbalanced life during the decade of their training are poorly qualified to teach their patients—or other medical students—about balanced living when they have not experienced this themselves.

Initiating change in medicine through political action

It was now 1970, and as the chief resident in internal medicine at Highland General Hospital, I'd had enough of the system. I stepped out and became the leader of the Highland Association of Interns and Residents, from which we coined the acronym *HAIR*. (You'll recall that in the '60s it was fashionable for men to have long hair.) We boldly decided to go on strike against our employer, Alameda County. Our chief grievance was that we were expected to work as many as 128 hours per week, sometimes for months at a time, and for meager compensation. Something needed to be done to change this outrageous policy.

HAIR won the local battle that year but didn't really win the war. The county agreed to shorten working hours and increase wages, but as I indicated, some of what was happening in 1970 still continues today. Nonetheless, it was empowering to know that we could stand up for what we believed in and make a difference. We also learned that we were largely on our own. We received little support from the teaching staff or from local physicians in private practice. In fact, many of them took an adversarial position. I remember receiving several threats that if I continued on the path I was taking, I might be dismissed from my residency program.

The themes of alienation and separation that got drummed into our heads during training were ingrained too deeply in our mentors for us to realistically expect political support from them. With a few notable exceptions, even those on our teaching staff whom we knew sympathized did not rally to support us. They too had been beaten by the system during their training and were too busy and tired themselves to muster the strength to take action in our behalf. I still believe that deep down inside, most of these physicians knew that the system needed to be changed. Yet, from another perspective, they also felt that they got through this training, so why shouldn't their students have to go through it, too? It's an irrational sentiment but understandably human.

Can physicians have their own union today?

Those of us in the early 1970s who rightly predicted that managed care, the brave new world of HMO medicine, was just around the corner—thereby guaranteeing that health care would soon become even further dominated by business values—realized that a physicians' union would be needed to protect wages, working conditions, and the quality of patient care. Shortly after our strike, the Union of American Physicians (UAP) was formed, and it still exists today.[5] While HAIR and the UAP had no formal affiliation, I believe that our strike helped spark the UAP's development.

Unfortunately, too few physicians have supported this potentially powerful organization, and today it has very limited power to initiate change. A mere 6 percent of American physicians belong to the UAP. Its membership is far too small to dictate policy for physicians, let alone for HMOs. However, this should not come as much of a surprise. How could a group of individuals who are trained to behave as "separatists" be expected to join together and form an effective union?

On the other hand, it is encouraging to watch the growth of Physicians for a National Health Program, a nonprofit activist organization of 16,000 physicians, medical students, and other health professionals who support single-payer national health insurance. We'll examine their progressive ideas about health care reform in chapter 9.

The next chapter returns us to the time of my paradigm-shattering discoveries in connection to Vicki's illness. By then, I had become a practicing physician in an environment increasingly in the grip of business values as well as a clash of paradigms. Little wonder that just a few years later, I was practically forced by circumstances to help pioneer an entirely new model of clinical practice.

Three

How "Scientific" Is Scientific Medicine?

It is simply no longer possible to believe much of the clinical research that is published, or to rely on the judgment of trusted physicians or authoritative medical guidelines. I take no pleasure in this conclusion, which I reached slowly and reluctantly over my two decades as an editor of The New England Journal of Medicine.

—Marcia Angell, *New York Review of Books,*
January 15, 2009

Sometime in my third decade as a successful practicing physician, I received a surprising call from the local office of the Medical Board of California.

"Is this Dr. Leonard Saputo?"

"Yes," I answered.

"This is the office of the California Medical Board. You are being advised to get an attorney. The California Medical Board is intending to revoke your license."

"For what?" I retorted, with a rising sense of shock.

"We are not required to provide that information to you at this time. However, we are demanding that you forward the chart [of the patient] to us immediately, or you will be fined $1,000 per day after one week for each day it is late."

I soon discovered what had happened: One of my patients had submitted a bill for the specialty tests I had ordered and it was summarily rejected.

Every insurance company has it own idiosyncratic version of what tests and procedures it will cover, and this company was no different. They did not understand what the tests were for, and rather than do some due diligence on the sound science behind my request, they had arbitrarily decided not to pay for the tests. When my patient informed me of this, I sent several letters to the company explaining that the patient was greatly improved because of the treatment that resulted from my having ordered the tests. I explained that the tests and the treatment weren't expensive, and that the insurer should indeed pay for them.

This patient was suffering from irritable bowel syndrome (IBS). He had needed a workup to find out why he had it, to determine its severity and to establish an effective treatment strategy. He had been to other physicians, who had followed the standard approaches designed to suppress his symptoms. These did not work very well and had also produced troubling side effects—which is why this man had come to me. I ordered two straightforward tests: a Comprehensive Digestive Stool Analysis (CDSA) and an intestinal permeability test. These led me to the correct treatment that solved his IBS symptoms.

Rather than listen to reason or at least engage in dialogue, this insurance company went straight to the Medical Board of California and informed the board that I'd ordered tests that they thought were not indicated. They further stated that this practice should be stopped immediately and that disciplinary action be administered. The Medical Board did in fact obtain a consultation from a general-practice professor at a local medical school. The professor had never heard of the tests, stated in his deposition that there could be no reasonable indication for doing them, and advised them to take punitive action.

What was occurring here was nothing short of a power struggle over what constitutes "good science" in the practice of medicine— and here was one representative case among thousands illustrating that, all too often, politics and even business determines what can be called legitimate science. Concealed at a deeper level is an even more severe clash between opposing scientific paradigms.

Meanwhile, my patient was delighted with the results of his treatment. Yet this was of no interest to the insurance company, the professor, or the Medical Board. No one even bothered to look into what the tests actually did or to appreciate that the laboratories doing the tests were approved by the federal government for quality assurance. No one was interested in looking at the scientific research underlying these tests. The Medical Board was skipping all that and was indeed intending to revoke my license to practice medicine forthwith!

I was forced to hire an attorney. Meanwhile, I also did some homework. It turned out that the Medical Board was offering continuing medical educational credits in several of their approved courses for physicians who wanted to learn about these very same cutting-edge tests that I had already incorporated into my medical practice! Today, these tests are mainstream and remain important in the diagnosis and management of IBS.

Of course, I won the case. But it cost me thousands of dollars to defend, and I was not able to recoup any part of these expenses because the Medical Board is protected by state law from either financial or personal injury recourse, whether right or wrong. The entire process took months of my time and caused considerable emotional distress for me, my office, and my family. As if this were not sufficient injustice, the Medical Board sidestepped the issue they initiated, citing me for having chart notes that were "not complete," and fined me $350 for this "misdemeanor." Apparently this tactic has been a common practice used when the Medical

Board wants to save face when they have lost a case. I never received an apology from the Medical Board, from the professor who provided an incompetent review of my case, or from the insurance company that reported me to the Medical Board. No action was taken against the insurance company or the general-practice professor providing incompetent testimony.

I tell this story because it illustrates what innovative physicians are up against when they face the power of politically aligned gatekeepers who are ignorant of the advances of medical science and are often profiting from the status quo—or who hold out against new science because of a dogmatic commitment to the reductionist disease care paradigm of mainstream medicine.[1]

My hospital rejects the science of clinical nutrition

As far back as the 12th century, the great Jewish medical philosopher Maimonides wrote, "Let nothing which can be treated by diet be treated by other means." This philosophy goes hand in hand with famous sayings of Hippocrates, "First, do no harm" and, as we noted earlier, "Let food be thy medicine and medicine be thy food."

Today, the discipline that inherited this ancient wisdom of Maimonides and Hippocrates—nutritional medicine—is an advanced science supported by thousands of peer-reviewed studies worldwide on every imaginable biomedical feature of every edible food or herb, as well as vitamins, minerals, and *nutraceuticals*—herbal extracts and other nutrients with curative properties. (In chapter 1, I introduced orthomolecular medicine, a refinement within this discipline.) When I naively attempted to develop a department of clinical nutrition at my local hospital that was based on the newest applications of this important science, I imagined that few would argue against nutrition's being particularly important for sick patients who had complex, varied, and increased nutritional demands.

I can certainly understand it when physicians oppose bringing untested scientific disciplines, medical tests, or procedures into a hospital; but it was almost incomprehensible to me that they would resist nutritional medicine and the orthomolecular medicine model I had first learned from Dr. Russ Jaffe. Yet my local hospital actually rejected, wholesale, my detailed proposal to do so in the late 1990s; indeed, this same hospital and most others reject clinical nutrition to this day. They continue to cling to the old disease care model—yet another sign of medical fundamentalism.

For those with even rudimentary knowledge of nutritional science, supporting optimal cellular function for every patient in the hospital is no more than common sense. Our cells have limitations in what they can do. They simply cannot manufacture energy and the important metabolic products our bodies need if they do not receive, through proper nutrition, the raw materials that are required to fuel these processes. This point is critical for two crucial reasons: Our metabolic needs increase when we are ill, and our cellular machinery may become limited in function because of illness.

Now, the first item on the agenda when it comes to providing good nutrition in hospitals is the questionable quality of hospital food itself. This is evidenced by the jokes one often hears about it and by numerous studies. One hard-to-believe survey of 200 hospitals with pediatric residency programs published in the December 2006 issue of the journal *Pediatrics* found that 59 of these hospitals had fast-food restaurants on-site![2]

This finding is appalling, of course. Even aside from our epidemic of childhood obesity, one would think that it would be a high priority to serve food in hospitals, especially to children, that is more nutrient dense than calorie dense, and that does not contain toxic trans fats, high-fructose corn syrup, or synthetic chemicals that the body must detoxify—all characteristics of the typical fast-food menu.

Aside from all that, hospital food should be *more* than nutritious. It should be savory and look delicious. It should be organically grown, be rich in healing herbs, and include the highest quality fruits, vegetables, and meats. All meals should be prepared by specially trained chefs who work under the supervision of herbalists and physician nutrition specialists. We should also be incorporating the culinary wisdom from great traditions such as Chinese medicine, Ayurveda, and Tibetan medicine.

But the reality is that hospitals have simply not been in the business of providing proper nutrition for critically ill hospitalized patients or children, who already have challenged diets. In part that's because the recommended daily requirements (Recommended Dietary Allowances, or RDAs) suggested by the U.S. Department of Agriculture (USDA)—which most hospitals follow—do not meet the needs of many healthy people, and this inadequate standard cannot be expected to provide the increased nutrition that sick patients require. To think so is simply bad science, despite the USDA's "official science" seal of approval, which is based at least in part on political and economic considerations.

In this connection, it is important to note that the Codex Alimentarius Commission, an intergovernmental body organized under the auspices of the United Nations, has long discussed the issue of creating international standards with regard to dietary supplements. If the Codex standards are adopted by the U.S.— which is possible in the next few years—the RDAs will be far below even our current therapeutic levels. According to the American Association for Health Freedom, a leading advocacy organization for integrative medicine, "Higher levels [than the new Codex RDA standards] would be considered 'drugs' and would be available only by prescription."

In order to provide optimal nutrition in hospitals, it would be necessary to serve fresh, whole, unprocessed, and unrefined foods that are free of toxic insecticides, pesticides, herbicides, preservatives, and additives—at a minimum. For more-advanced nutritional therapy, many hospitalized patients also need what is known as *parenteral* (intravenous) nutrition, an approach that requires the supervision of a physician specially trained in cellular biochemistry who may give nutrient dosages that are hundreds and in certain situations even thousands of times higher than the minimum RDAs.

Our bodies have enough trouble detoxifying the polluted food, water, and air that we consume under normal circumstances on a daily basis, let alone handling the toxins in processed foods served in our hospitals. When we are sick and our toxic loads are even higher, our ability to detoxify may become critically challenged and lead to significant worsening of illness.

We've noted that detoxification is another sophisticated science that is out of favor in mainstream medicine. Yet it too deserves special attention, particularly in people who are ill. For example, liver detoxification is critically important when pharmaceuticals are being used on sick patients, yet most clinicians overlook this issue. A great deal of new research is published in our scientific literature but still not included in medical training or in clinical practice. What the science of nutritional medicine has taught us in this arena is vital, and it is indefensible that it is not a major part of every patient's hospital care. The sad truth is that our dietitians and gastroenterologists get only the barest exposure to this kind of training.

To summarize, there is room for vast improvement in providing specialized foods, food extracts, herbs, and other supplements that can support the metabolic needs of our cells. In addition, we need to provide patients with more support for detoxification, and in particular be more proactive in fostering through natural or noninvasive means the gastrointestinal tract's central role in digesting and absorbing what we ingest and in eliminating toxins. In the critically ill, all of these factors are even more important to consider.

With this as background, let's return to the story of my attempt to start a department of clinical nutrition at my hospital. I did my homework in this case as well: First, I managed to find a well-qualified candidate to chair this proposed new department. He was retiring as a professor of medicine from a nearby medical school and had extensive specialized training in clinical nutrition; and, to my great surprise, he was interested in affiliating with a local hospital. I then started the process of determining how to structure the department within the bylaws of my hospital's administration. I presented our concept at a general meeting of the department of medicine, and most of my colleagues responded by agreeing that it was worth exploring further.

I was invited to explain the idea to a subcommittee that had ultimate decision-making power. To my amazement, this committee reached a unanimous agreement that there was no reason to expand the nutritional expertise at our hospital! The reason given was that we already had dietitians and gastroenterologists who had long been providing these services and were "doing just fine." In their view, the hospital had gotten along quite well without making health care any more complicated and expensive than it already was.

It is even more remarkable that the dietitians and gastroenterologists themselves did not welcome the expertise of a specialist trained in nutritional medicine to help them support their patients. If anyone would know the limitations of their services and their training, you'd think it would be them! It made me wonder if I had naively stumbled into the middle of a battle of egos or an economic turf war rather than a process oriented toward simply trying to improve the care of our patients.

Because of the fundamentalist commitment of medical training to the disease care paradigm, gastroenterologists are not trained experts in nutrition—or, for that matter, detoxification. They are experts in diagnosing and treating gastrointestinal diseases using mainstream medical technologies, pharmaceutical drugs, and established treatment protocols. And while registered dietitians do their best to provide for the caloric needs and general metabolic support for hospitalized patients, they are not trained as physicians and shouldn't even attempt to manage the therapeutic intricacies involved in providing the complex metabolic support required by the seriously ill.

While I was disappointed, I wasn't really surprised. As I look back, it is easy to understand what had happened. My colleagues were no different than I was prior to Vicki's illness. Until just a few short years earlier, I too had been convinced that the practice of medicine was near perfect and that we understood nutritional medicine quite well. I truly believed that we had a tremendous volume of information on nutrition that was evidence based and that we were the best-trained people on the planet to manage the "relatively minimal" nutritional needs of people who were sick. I too was stuck in an outdated paradigm, blinded by a narrow system of belief that confers on its adherents the uncanny ability to filter out an entire branch of evidence-based science!

It was also a question of sheer ignorance and naiveté: The fact that any physician could believe that he had mastered the complexities of managing nutritional therapies for hospitalized patients when he had a mere two hours of training in medical school in basic nutrition is indeed remarkable. Ironically, at the time I was trying to introduce nutritional medicine to my hospital, more than 25 teaching medical centers throughout the United States were offering specialized degrees for "physician nutrition specialists." These specialists were being trained for an additional one to two years beyond residency training in such fields as internal medicine, endocrinology, and pediatrics.

Additional mundane factors must have made it easy for the medical staff at our hospital to reject the introduction of a department of clinical nutrition. Medicine, though a healing art, is also a business. The factor of underlying turf war issues that could affect who would control certain health care services and their related financial rewards never overtly surfaced. Yet it doesn't take much insight to recognize that the turf of every field of medicine pursued in this hospital, not just gastroenterology and dietitics, would have been impacted by a department of clinical nutrition.

Individuals whose income might be jeopardized are not generally receptive to changing the status quo. And, of course, market share for certain types of hospital services might have decreased if this new department had been created. Finally, adding a bit more insult to injury, some insurers did not (and still do not) cover services rendered by a department of clinical nutrition.

Ideally, a healer would not be influenced by economic factors when it came to caring for patients. Yet we live in a fundamentally materialistic culture, and business is still business, even in the "sacred" medical profession.

A hospital pharmacy blocks an essential and scientifically proven nutrient

I continued my effort to bring nutritional medicine to our hospital, hoping that my persistence—even on a much smaller scale this time—would eventually create change. However, this turned out to be yet another exercise in futility.

A few months later, I still hadn't given up. I made a request to the hospital pharmacy committee that the supplement coenzyme Q10 (CoQ10) be added to its formulary. It made sense to begin with a supplement that had been researched in the mainstream peer-reviewed medical literature and offered clear, important, and safe benefits for certain patients.

Coenzyme Q10 is a plant-derived, vitamin-like substance that has many important applications that are useful and safe in medical practice. It is essential for normal energy production by most cells of our body, is a powerful antioxidant, and improves heart function in nearly every measurable parameter when it is given to people with low serum levels. It has also been reported to have a role in the prevention and treatment of certain kinds of cancer and has been used to slow the progression of Parkinson's disease.

One of the saddest oversights regarding the lack of usage of coenzyme Q10 is that several published scientific studies show that it can prevent the commonly associated cardiac toxicity of the chemotherapy drug Adriamycin, which can cause a lethal cardiomyopathy. It is such a shame that a nutrient with no known toxicity is not at least tried, especially given the possibility of life-threatening congestive heart failure that sometimes can occur along with this cancer treatment. What is there to lose by giving it a try?

It is well known that certain medications such as the *statin* drugs, which are almost universally used to lower cholesterol, interfere with the production of coenzyme Q10. This makes it even more important to use in patients whose metabolism is challenged by statin drugs, particularly if they are also taking Adriamycin or have an illness in which energy production is compromised. And in an article published in the *American Journal of Cardiology* in June 2007, it was shown that coenzyme Q10 reduced the muscle pain caused by statin drugs by 40 percent in 16 of 18 patients studied and that it improved their quality of life.[3] It would seem that for this reason alone, adding this nutrient to the hospital pharmaceutical armamentarium would be eagerly supported.

I asked for permission to attend a pharmacy committee meeting to formally present my request and was pleased when I received the invitation. When I arrived, to my surprise, about 15 people were in attendance, far more than the usual three to five people who attended these routine meetings. I thought, "Great, there is at least some interest in nutritional medicine." I was correct. There was a lot of interest, but not the kind I had hoped for.

Everyone listened to the evidence I shared from mainstream, alternative, and nutritional medical journals, and I felt encouraged by their receptivity. No one contested anything during the presentation. It seemed like a slam-dunk, and that coenzyme Q10 would soon find itself in the hospital formulary.

To my shock, the proposal was unanimously rejected. The treatment was "too new," and even though it might be a reasonable addition, the pharmacy committee did not want to include it in the formulary until more substantiating information was published in a greater number of conventional medical journals. It is interesting that since then, many major hospitals now include coenzyme Q10 in their drug formularies. When I checked back a few months ago, I found that it is finally in my hospital's formulary.

The hospital pharmacy continued to privately allow me to order coenzyme Q10, and they supplied all of my patients with the dosages ordered. Perhaps they respected my use of this nutrient, but I was never sure that their real motivation wasn't related to avoiding a potential legal nightmare if—after I had ordered coenzyme Q10 for a patient—it was not given, and the patient suffered a consequence.

Issues like this make it frustrating for physicians who have gone out of their way to study and learn how to use new therapies, and then find themselves stymied by dogma and its associated resistance to change, arrogance, ignorance, and turf wars related to power and money. It is almost incomprehensible that so many physicians simply do not regard nutrition as important in restoring and maintaining good health when so much good, solid scientific evidence supports its value, especially now that we are in an era of public awakening to the fact that nutrition is critical to good health.

In the end, it comes down once again to a war of paradigms. While optimal nutrition and orthomolecular medicine belong squarely in the emerging integral-health medicine paradigm, these things are barely given lip service in the prevailing disease care model, which focuses on a battle against nature rather than on preventing illness or restoring health by supporting wellness. This worldview clash guarantees that as long as physicians who use nutrition as the basis for preventing or treating illness are in the minority paradigm, and regardless of the scientific evidence for their positions, there will be a particular prejudice against them. As a result, many outstanding, pioneering physicians have lost their licenses and as a result had to relocate to more open-minded states such as Arizona, New Mexico, Nevada, and Washington.[4]

I face resistance in bringing forward a proven technology

It is one thing for a hospital to refuse to carry nutritional supplements. It is another and far more serious matter when a breakthrough in medicine is suppressed by competing businesses or lack of physician interest due to prejudice, cynicism, or a case of paradigm clash. Think about it: Every time a new technology comes along that is superior to an old one, what happens to the old technology? It's phased out, of course. But who wants to have some aspect of their business phased out when it means taking a financial hit? Might it be to their personal financial advantage to suppress this innovation?

Well, suppression happens all the time. Allow me to present just one egregious case.

How would you feel if there were an inexpensive, safe, simple, and highly effective treatment for easing pain and speeding up healing by about 50 percent, but it was not yet approved by the U.S. Food and Drug Administration (FDA), which was ignoring it? Could this be because of a conspiracy against the technology? What if there were good research behind the new treatment, and yet mainstream medical journals made ridiculous excuses for refusing to publish it?

Have I piqued your interest yet?

Further, could there be such an all-encompassing conspiracy resulting in millions of people continuing to suffer needlessly because they were being deprived of a treatment that could reduce or eliminate the need for drugs? Would the makers of more than 40 blockbuster drugs object if these drugs were no longer in such high demand? And if all this were actually happening, would you not be morally outraged? Let me tell you an amazing personal story, and let's see what you think.

In 1999, I contacted an electrical engineer named Maurice Bales after reading an ad that his company, Bales Scientific, had placed in a medical journal. The ad seemed a bit outrageous in its claims, and I was about to toss the journal into the wastebasket when I noticed that his phone number was local. Curious, I called him. Maurice said he had invented a device, called a *photon stimulator*, that emitted near-infrared light of a certain frequency, which, he claimed, could relieve most kinds of pain. I didn't believe him at first. If what he was claiming was correct, then why wasn't something this impressive already being used in clinical practice?

Yet Maurice seemed honest. And he wasn't trying to sell me anything; he only wanted the chance to show me that it worked and see what I thought. He invited me to bring patients suffering from pain to his office for a free demonstration. Reluctantly, I agreed. I didn't have time to waste on something I suspected was much overrated, but I *was* curious, and if somehow he was correct, I wanted to know about it.

I invited two patients with severe pain to try the treatment. One had multiple sclerosis (MS) and was for the most part bedridden with pain and unable to walk without crutches. The other patient had a ruptured lumbar disc that was causing intractable pain in his low back. To my shock, both patients were substantially improved in just one 15-minute treatment with Maurice's light! Over the next couple of weeks, the man with MS remained in far less pain after a total of eight treatments. He was up out of bed most of the day, could walk more upright, and even returned to full-time work. The treatments did not change the overall progression of his disease process, but for a year he was much improved and was very appreciative. The other patient had significant but only temporary relief of his symptoms after a similar number of treatments.

I was by now becoming captivated by Maurice's technology. For the next three months, he invited me bring two or three of my patients to his office after work from 5 to 7 p.m. on Mondays, Wednesdays, and Fridays. These patients had a wide variety of painful conditions that included disc problems, carpal tunnel syndrome, tennis elbow, sports and other traumatic injuries, neuropathic pain, headaches, TMJ problems (inflammation of the joint that connects the jaw to the skull), and much more. The device worked to some degree on each one! By the end of this period, I began to expect that almost anyone with pain would be helped by Maurice's "magic" light. Maurice thereupon generously set me up with a lot of expensive equipment so that I could help people and also bring the technology forward. He was passionate about disseminating his light therapy, but I was the only MD he could persuade to try it. In fact, today, with only a few exceptions, I still am. Of course, being a minority of one hasn't stopped me.

Over a decade, my practice in pain management treatment has grown to the point that it now consumes about half of my time. Along the way, Maurice also coached me regarding the importance of using varying combinations of other adjunctive disciplines, such as physical therapy, many styles of bodywork, chiropractic, guided imagery, acupuncture, psychology, and applied kinesiology, in conjunction with near-infrared light therapy through photonic stimulation. Since we got started with this work in 1999, I have treated literally thousands of patients. The vast majority are very appreciative of what this technology has done for them, and they have enthusiastically referred many of their friends to become my patients.

How do the photons work? In the simplest terms, they excite electrons within the energy-producing mitochondria of cells in injured tissues. This process is thought to enable these cells to increase their production of ATP, the energy currency of our cells, and thereby stimulate the return of more normal cellular physiology. An additional effect is increased blood flow to injured tissues, which promotes both pain relief and faster healing.

Finally, as a pioneering physician using photonic stimulation, I felt compelled to go the next step. In 2004, Maurice and I, and a few others at the Health Medicine Center, self-funded a clinical trial on 120 patients suffering from advanced painful diabetic neuropathy, a debilitating condition. The trial was carried out at the VA Medical Center in nearby Martinez, California. Our team included ten experts in pain management, who provided a variety of contributions to the study, including specific research tools. Our objective was to show that only four treatments of seven minutes each on four successive days using photonic stimulation could relieve pain, improve sensation, and improve balance.

These patients with severe diabetic neuropathy had been among the most difficult to manage with conventional treatment. Most were routinely treated with pharmaceuticals such as narcotics, NSAIDs (nonsteroidal anti-inflammatory drugs), Neurontin, and antidepressants, which often had severe side effects such as sleepiness, nausea, weakness, and a variety of digestive symptoms.

Many of our 120 subjects had multiple additional causes of pain, such as disc disease, vascular insufficiency, poisoning from Agent Orange or heavy metals, and alcoholism. Yet most of them still improved, their pain having either disappeared or been greatly reduced. Also, the sensitivity on the bottom of their feet was increased, their balance was improved, and their overall quality of life was better. And these results came after just a single week of treatment. Patients with mild neuropathy that I treated for so many years in my office have been much easier to help. After a short treatment regimen, most of these patients' milder symptoms disappear for months to years!

A scientific article that I coauthored with VA Medical Center physicians and University of California, San Francisco (UCSF)

School of Medicine researchers showed conclusively that photonic stimulation is a valuable tool in treating people with diabetic neuropathy. In many ways, this was an unprecedented result: I can't think of any new medical device that does so much for such a small investment of time, money, and expertise, especially when compared with the alternatives that are now used in clinical practice. Our article, which lays out this startling evidence, has been presented to many relevant medical journals over a period of two years, but with no success. Their excuses for not publishing it have originated from either their total lack of understanding of the technology and an unwillingness to learn it, or what amounts to an unscientific bias that categorically denies that it could have benefits for our patients.

The FDA has also refused to consider giving Maurice Bales approval for the technology's use in the treatment of any aspect of what our study showed, despite our strong data, the obvious safety of the device, and the device's amazing cost-effectiveness. Could this coincide with purported severe management problems at the FDA's division that handles medical devices? The Associated Press reported on January 8, 2009, that a group of federal scientists sent the Obama administration "an unusual blunt letter" complaining that FDA managers squelch scientific debate in this division, alleging that top FDA managers "committed the most outrageous misconduct by ordering, coercing and intimidating FDA physicians and scientists . . . to go along."[5]

Whatever the case, it is not legal for Maurice or me to claim that this device works for the treatment of diabetic neuropathy—although I am permitted to use it without advertising, as with any other "off label" treatment. I don't make specific claims to the public, but I have a constant stream of patients who are happy with the results. I feel a considerable amount of satisfaction when I offer as part of my practice photonic stimulation for a wide range of painful conditions, especially when it's supplemented by the work of other practitioners in my integrative clinic.

This may lead you, as it has me, to wonder: Through word of mouth by my patients and my own efforts to spread the word over the last ten years, many doctors in my region know about this technology. Yet why haven't any of them referred their patients to me for treatment, especially when no other option exists than to use a cocktail of toxic drugs that have innumerable side effects? There are several reasons, none of which are very satisfying.

First of all, most physicians, especially those in HMO medicine, are simply too busy treating patients; they lack the needed time to pay attention to ideas that are not yet in the mainstream, not to mention new findings that appear in mainstream medical journals. Second, physicians have actually become leery of pretty much all mainstream scientific information, *let alone* alternative approaches; Marcia Angell's quote at the top of this chapter is beginning to typify the reigning attitude. Finally, they distrust colleagues who seem to have become preoccupied with any unconventional treatment. They are particularly skeptical if there is any possibility of a financial conflict of interest. All these attitudes are understandable, but unfortunately they can lead to the suppression of some new technologies that are important.

Ten years have now passed, yet this revolutionary technology is *still* not in mainstream medicine. At first, I had no idea that people would resist this information because it sounded too good to be true or that some might even actively interfere with its advancement into clinical practice because of economic conflict of interest.

Yet, photonic stimulation is good, and it is true. Several of my patients have had what should be considered miraculous cures from their pain. One patient, for example, with AIDS had been treated with conventional antiretroviral therapy and as a complication developed a lymphoma. He was treated for the lymphoma with chemotherapy. In yet another complication of this treatment, he developed a very painful condition called *osteonecrosis* throughout the bones in his body. He was being managed by a pain clinic and was on large doses of narcotics and a multitude of other drugs. Nonetheless, he was incapacitated with pain and could not work. This man heard about the light treatment from a friend and decided to try it. In just a single 15-minute treatment with Maurice's light, his pain cleared and has never returned. We were both in tears over the excitement of what had happened in just minutes for a condition that had become chronic and incapacitating. Amazingly, I never got a call from a single one of his doctors—neither his AIDS physician nor his pain management team; none of them cared to ask what I had done to help this poor man. I describe other such cases later in the book.

My experience with photonic stimulation technology is not an isolated instance; an amazing array of other suppressed technologies and natural treatments—all backed by strong science and overwhelming evidence like ours—are also covered in many other books. The wheels turn slowly when one is up against those with a financial commitment to a fatally narrow set of tools and concepts. It can be especially egregious when you are the purveyor of a simple, obvious remedy that has the potential to upstage and even make obsolete billion-dollar enterprises.

Just how evidence based is today's medicine?

Still, there is much hope. Even within the narrow paradigm that now prevails, many brilliant high-tech scientific achievements are able to filter through the inertia and resistance of the modern medical establishment. We have accomplished the almost unimaginable feat of uncovering the human genome and are now on the brink of making advances in stem cell research that promise to revolutionize the practice of medicine. It is almost unbelievable that modern science has developed the technical skill to change the genetics of a cell and control its metabolic function. Because of advances like these, we may one day be able to reverse chronic diseases such as cancer, congestive heart failure, strokes, Parkinson's disease, MS, diabetes, and many others. It may not be unreasonable to believe that the slow process of scientific discovery could someday expose the mysteries of illness and make it possible to eliminate many horrible diseases.

This exciting research notwithstanding, just how scientific is the medicine being practiced in the average clinical setting today?

In 1978, a report by the Congressional Office of Technology Assessment concluded, "No more than fifteen percent of medical interventions are supported by reliable scientific evidence."[6] Thirteen years later, in 1991, Richard Smith, editor of the prestigious *British Medical Journal*, came to the same conclusion. He went on to comment that "only one percent of the articles in medical journals are scientifically sound and partly because many treatments have not been assessed at all."[7] And David Grimes, MD, stated in the 1993 issue of the *Journal of the American Medical Association* (*JAMA*) that "much, if not most, of contemporary medical practice still lacks a scientific foundation."[8] Houston, we have a problem!

Of course, scientific method requires that we test any and all claims or new discoveries through the use of clinical trials. Conducting research that is randomized, double blind, placebo controlled, and crossed over is the very stuff of genuine modern-day science. Unfortunately, scientists and their sponsors have not always applied this tried-and-true methodology in a way that was scrupulous, careful, or even honest. One indicator of the problem is that too many conflicting outcomes emanate from different laboratories or teams of scientists who are studying the same issues. What on earth causes such large discrepancies in results? How is one to know where the truth lies?

Further, in too many cases, short-term and incomplete studies are used as the primary or sole basis for clinical treatment protocols. As we will further explore in chapter 5, this tendency to use shortcuts for getting new drugs or procedures to market has led to the adoption of many dubious treatments that have later been removed from clinical practice because of adverse and sometimes lethal side effects.

The problem is also easily traced to conflicts of interest, usually involving relationships between researchers in universities and the sponsors funding their studies. The amount of money spent by industry in medical research and development was nearly $60 billion in 2000, or 60 percent of the overall total that year, far greater than the roughly $25 billion spent by the federal government. Today, about *70 percent* of all funding for clinical drug trials originates from the pharmaceutical industry itself. Remember, these are the folks whose products are supposedly being objectively and scientifically tested!

It is not uncommon for drug companies to "supervise" the studies they fund at universities, giving them the right to determine what gets published. They reserve the prerogative to write the summaries of the articles, rather than the scientists who did the research. In fact, in some published research articles, the principal investigator had nothing to do with the study except to allow her name to be used—for a fee.

In January 2007, Harvard researchers published an article in the *PLoS Medicine* online journal, published by the Public Library of Science, that considered the influence of those who paid for a particular study on the outcome of the study.[9] They reviewed 111 studies, some paid for by independent groups, the rest funded by industry. They reported these results:

- Industry-funded studies were 400 to 800 percent more likely to favor industry interests.

- Thirty-eight percent of independently funded studies ran against the interests of the funder.

Consider, in addition, this article published in the January 20, 2007, issue of the *British Medical Journal,* titled, "What Have We Learnt from Vioxx?" The lead author, Harlan M. Krumholz, the Harold H. Hines, Jr., Professor of Medicine at Yale University, claimed that the pharmaceutical company Merck had not only obscured critical data on the drug's toxicity, but had also given a biased presentation of its research and had used ghostwriters to author papers on it. He went on to state that "its [Merck's] behavior may not be any different from that of others in the pharmaceutical or biotechnology industry." Vioxx, as you may remember, was withdrawn from the market in 2004 after massive litigation and a media uproar resulted when this drug, used as a painkiller worldwide, was linked to many thousands of heart attacks, cardiac deaths, and strokes.[10]

Dozens of other cases are almost as blatant. In 2001, for example, TAP Pharmaceuticals pled guilty and agreed to pay $875 million to settle criminal and civil charges brought under the False Claims Act over its fraudulent marketing of Lupron, a drug used for treatment of cancer.[11] To get a sense of proportion, contrast this with the evidence for the use of vitamin D as a cancer deterrent. Almost 90 scientific studies over many decades have shown that vitamin D is the cancer-protective factor generated from direct contact with sunlight, reducing cancer risk by up to 50 percent. A definitive, carefully controlled study published in 2007 on the effect of 1,000 IU/day of vitamin D (with calcium) on cancer incidence showed, after four years, that the cancer risk was 60 percent lower than with a placebo, and 77 percent lower when corrected for participants who had already had cancers present.[12] Other studies have shown equally significant associations of vitamin D with the reduction of diabetes, number of falls by the elderly, MS, and other maladies. Yet, as with the case of the simple technology of photonic stimulation, how much have you heard about this astounding scientific evidence?

A few more crucial points: Randomized, double-blind, placebo-controlled trials are not the only way to validate treatments for clinical practice. Traditional systems such as those in Chinese, Tibetan, and Native American medicine are all time tested and have strong empirical value, whether they are tested "scientifically" or not; they have endured for hundreds or even thousands of years for a reason. Nonetheless, as in the case of acupuncture, strict scientific study has progressed greatly in recent years, even as experts debate the proper research methodology to be used to correct for disparities in the skill of a given practitioner and for related variables.

Finally, it should be noted that the scientific method as conventionally applied in medical research strives to measure the effect of a *single* factor, often a drug or technology, on a symptom or disease. While this approach can provide essential data, often multiple factors are involved in causing illness, and many aspects of our physiology must be addressed in providing an effective treatment. For this reason, a new clinical research model has emerged that is called an *outcome* study. In these studies, many treatment modalities are simultaneously varied, and the cumulative effect of different sets of variables is measured over time. For example, an integrative physician treating a patient with cancer might seek to simultaneously strengthen the patient's immunity with supplements and herbs; alkalinize his pH; support the ability of his gut to digest, absorb, and detoxify what is eaten; add high-dose antioxidants; and start him on a regimen of exercise and yoga. If in controlled clinical trials the patients on this protocol improved, we'd know the outcome but not the roles of each of the factors in modifying the course of the illness.

Ethics issues for research scientists and the FDA

Next up is the issue of professional ethics among some medical research scientists. In a July 2006 article titled, "Stop Misbehaving," Ushma S. Neill, executive editor of the eminent *Journal of Clinical Investigation*, wrote, "Scientists are usually thought to be beyond reproach, but with the recent spate of high-profile ethical transgressions by scientists, the public's trust in science and scientists is deteriorating. The numerous cases of scientific misconduct that have crossed my desk in the last year leave me disenchanted, disappointed, and disillusioned."[13]

Of course, most scientists are honest and operate with the highest integrity. Yet every year, a surprising number of scientific medical articles are published that are later found to have been falsified. This kind of ethical misconduct is often related to conflicts of interest involving financial gain, career advancement, and personal fame.

Pharmaceutical companies are in business to further the interests of their investors, but doctors and medical schools have no such excuse: Their only responsibility is to patients. "The mission of medical schools and teaching hospitals—and what justifies their tax-exempt status—is to educate the next generation of physicians, carry out scientifically important research, and care for the sickest members of society," wrote former *New England Journal of Medicine* (*NEJM*) editor-in-chief Marcia Angell. "It is not to enter into lucrative commercial alliances with the pharmaceutical industry. As reprehensible as many industry practices are, I believe the behavior of much of the medical profession is even more culpable."[14]

One might claim that we have one final bulwark against an industry riddled with conflicts of interest and the commercial drive for profit—federal government regulation. So, can we trust the FDA to safeguard clinical trials of new drugs and devices to make sure they are conducted properly? It is an appalling but well-known fact that many FDA officials also engage in financial relationships with pharmaceutical and/or technology companies. No wonder more than four of five Americans surveyed believe that the FDA makes decisions influenced by politics rather than medical science. In fact, in a study published in *JAMA* in October 2006, this very subject was addressed.[15] Of nearly 3,000 FDA panel members who were anonymously interviewed, the study reported that 28 percent disclosed a financial relationship within the previous year either with the company that made a drug under discussion or with a competitor. The most common ties were consulting arrangements, research contracts or grants, and stock holdings or other investments.

In response to harsh criticism from Congress and the press after a myriad of scandals—most involving its approvals of drugs like Vioxx and Lupron that have cost untold tens of thousands of lives—FDA commissioner Dr. Edward von Eschenbach convened a special internal committee of inquiry that included several outside experts to assess whether the FDA is actually able to accomplish its mission. Its final report, issued early in 2008, titled, *FDA Science and Mission at Risk*, stated, "*The FDA cannot fulfill its mission because its scientific base has eroded and its scientific organizational structure is weak* [emphasis added]." It went on to state that "its scientific workforce does not have sufficient capacity and capability." Amazingly, it further stated, "The FDA science agenda lacks a coherent structure and vision, as well as effective coordination and prioritization." And among the shocking conclusions was this one: "The FDA does not have the capacity to ensure the safety of food for the nation."[16]

Well, at least one government agency has the honesty to indict itself for its own incompetence! But again, how many Americans or even members of Congress have *heard* about this self-indictment?

It is notable that as a result of the erroneous assumption that mainstream medicine truly is science driven, evidence based, and properly regulated, physicians have held all other nonmainstream health care disciplines to standards of research that they often do not realize are far more rigorous than those to which they hold themselves. Physicians have all but ignored the salient fact that many traditional health care disciplines, notably Chinese medicine and Ayurvedic medicine, have been validated over untold generations of trial and error. Their continued use for billions of people in many parts of the world today is a strong testimonial that they do work. Plus, these and other non-Western medical disciplines have also been subject to rigorous scientific scrutiny as these cultures have evolved their own scientific establishments and peer-reviewed medical journals.

Competing scientific models for
defining disease and determining treatment

A famous old argument between two well-known nineteenth-century scientists, Pasteur and Beauchamp, still goes on today: What is the most important factor in determining whether or not we will get sick or die when we are exposed to a microbe? Is it the external invading microbe itself, or is it the internal defenses of the body—or lack thereof—that make the most difference? High-tech medicine, following Louis Pasteur, has clearly taken the former position. Its signature activity is that of killing off the microbe, knocking out the cancer, and in general battling the invasion of any and all disease by means of drugs, technology, and surgery. And in a sense, its reigning attitude—as we have noted—is that of a *war against nature herself.* This approach focuses on looking outside of ourselves to find solutions rather than looking inside.

Opposing this view, Antoine Beauchamp, a scientific contemporary of Pasteur's, argued that an unbalanced lifestyle, stress, a poor diet, and the like make us vulnerable to disease, and that we can protect ourselves by strengthening our natural defenses in those places where we have become vulnerable. Beauchamp completely rejected Pasteur's ideas and put forward the thesis that our "biological terrain" is the cause of disease; it was Beauchamp who proclaimed, "The primary cause of disease is in us, always in us."

Clearly, both perspectives are important and deserve attention. The former approach searches desperately for magic bullets that can attack disease from the outside. The second focuses on strengthening our inner defenses so that we are less vulnerable to illness in the first place. Yet it's clear that Pasteur's prejudice fits much more neatly into a culture in which people prefer to shirk responsibility for their own health.

In the emerging new model of medicine, we are awakening to the fact that primary care should not be focused merely on treating disease from the outside. In an ideal health care system, we would rarely get sick in the first place, because the central objective would be to focus *on the inside*—following Beauchamp—to maintain wellness and vitality through prevention and a strong focus on natural defenses. This, again, is what I call true and sustainable *health care*, as opposed to *disease care.*

It can't be stated too often: The cornerstone of a reasonable system of true health care is healthy lifestyle. We have noted that this includes eating a healthy diet, getting enough exercise and sleep, avoiding stress, maintaining a healthy weight, avoiding toxic exposures, supporting detoxification—and perhaps most important of all, having a meaningful purpose in life.

Neither Pasteur nor Beauchamp was entirely right or wrong. They were simply pointing to different ends of a spectrum that explains how we get sick or remain healthy. Healthy lifestyle is on one end of the spectrum, and germs and other factors that "attack" the body are on the other. It is hard to imagine that anyone today would argue against the premise that both factors usually play a role in causing illness. And this insight is at the root of today's evolving concepts within the new discipline that I now call integral-health medicine, which methodically integrates insights about both the inner world and the outer environment of the patient, as each is conditioned by its economic, social, and cultural context.

Most laypersons are unaware that medicine has only a limited understanding of the causes of most chronic diseases; as a result, doctors can rarely direct their mighty high-tech weapons to a definite target. This shortcoming has left the door open for the new, integrally informed model of medicine. As we will see in later chapters, this hybrid approach focuses on the premise that the body itself does the healing and that medicine should support this process as its top priority—but that the disinterested scientific search for technologies and drugs that can make people feel better still has a place.

Cellular health: a key concept underlying the new science of medicine

Over the past 40 years, the paradigm more in line with Beauchamp's position has been gaining momentum. The importance of lifestyle factors, and the recognition of the body's innate wisdom concerning its own natural healing abilities, are just now beginning to emerge into mainstream thinking. Again, this approach is focused primarily on strengthening the defenses of the body rather than fighting what has "attacked" the body and created malfunction and disease.

According to the model I have adopted, the scientific core of this approach involves four main factors, and each is addressed at the cellular level:

- Nutritional needs of our cells

- Elimination of toxic substances

- Genetic defects

- Psychospiritual factors

As surprising and simplistic as it may seem, a great deal of research and clinical observation has shown that varied combinations of these four factors are *always* the basis for the cause of *every* disease. It is impossible to fall sick if all your cells are functioning perfectly. Let's look at each of these factors in more detail.

The imperative of properly nourishing our bodies

Consider that each individual human cell is analogous to a microscopic industrial plant. It requires a steady supply of a wide range of raw materials to manufacture the nutrients required for structural maintenance and the production of hormones, enzymes, energy, and so on, to keep the body functioning smoothly and efficiently. We've noted that a cell simply cannot manufacture these important substances unless it has the proper and continuous supply of all the raw materials it needs. This is why what we eat is so important.

Yet it is not sufficient to simply supply the body with foods that contain the nutrients required to produce all the chemicals it needs. In order to remain healthy, the body must also be able to digest, absorb, metabolize, transport, and when necessary, detoxify what is consumed. We are not just what we eat—we are what we eat, absorb, deliver, and utilize at the cellular level. And many processes must be intact for this to happen correctly.

These factors highlight why it is so critically important to address nutrition in everyone, whether to restore or maintain optimal health. It is also important to appreciate that we all have different needs because of variations in our *biochemical individuality*. This means that because of our genetic makeup, some people will need far more of a certain nutrient than others; in fact, this may vary as much as 20-fold in some cases. As we have noted, this becomes especially important in people who are sick and have increased nutrient demands plus decreased capacity to detoxify.

Most of us do not appreciate the extent of the nutritional deficiencies that exist in the standard American diet. As we migrated from the country—where we consumed nature's fresh, whole, unprocessed, and unrefined foods—to the city, where there is a large population that needs to be fed and cannot easily grow its own food, we were faced with new problems that have made it difficult to easily provide enough food to feed everyone. Transportation, packaging, processing, and storage were suddenly new and important challenges.

We responded by developing a sophisticated technology to mass-produce crops and increase their yield by using pesticides, herbicides, and fertilizers. Then we added a number of chemicals that had never before been in a human body, in order to refine, process, and store foods for prolonged periods of time. As this technology grew, we began creating "foods" that are so deficient in nutrients and so full of synthetic chemicals that many of them can no longer accurately be called real food. Nonetheless, they store well, taste good, feed massive populations that cannot provide their own food, and are good for business.

These highly processed foods are generally high in calories and low in nutrient density. It should not be surprising that these commercialized food products have led to a pandemic of both obesity and malnutrition, which can even occur in the same person. The USDA has done at least three studies (known as the NHANES, for National Health and Nutrition Examination Surveys) on tens of thousands of people over the past 30 years and has documented that the standard American diet, or SAD, is just that, "sad."[17, 18] You don't have to look for the nutritional deficiencies in third world countries to find malnutrition. There is an underappreciated epidemic right here in America today, and according to our own scientific studies, nearly everyone is affected to some extent.

What about supplements to compensate for the SAD diet? You may be surprised that under circumstances such as those in California, where all of us have easy access to fresh, inexpensive, and especially organic foods, I do not recommend taking supplements—not even vitamin pills. I don't perceive supplements to be any different from pharmaceutical drugs except that they are hundreds of thousands of times safer. However, if we eat a healthy diet, exercise, get eight hours a sleep every night, maintain a reasonable weight, and don't suffer from excessive stress, then I don't believe we need them.

I also believe that most of us don't need to supplement with antioxidants either. Our bodies have a remarkable, though admittedly limited, ability to adapt to the increased free-radical stress that results from both toxic exposures and exercise. During hard exercise, we produce enormous amounts of free radicals, which are byproducts of energy production in the mitochondria of our cells. However, our natural antioxidant defense system can and does adapt to these increased levels of free radicals by making more antioxidants itself. If we take antioxidants in the form of supplements, we remove the body's need to make them, and when we need to produce them at times when we are vulnerable, a serious lag time can result. Although extremely minor when compared with the hazards of most pharmaceuticals, overdosing with some vitamins and antioxidants can be dangerous. For example, excessive levels of vitamin A can cause osteoporosis. High levels of vitamin E can increase mortality in patients with congestive heart failure. And overuse of vitamin C can cause severe anemia in people with a genetic blood disorder called G6PD deficiency.

That said, I do practice medicine by relying more on lifestyle management and the judicious use of natural, noninvasive remedies and dietary supplements than on invasive therapies. By supporting the body's biochemistry, we can often correct problems that led to its disease; and nearly always this approach is far safer than using pharmaceutical drugs. Yet there is a time and place for all treatment styles.

Finally, we have one more factor to contend with in these times: the rising cost of food and food staples. A study published in the *Journal of the American Dietetic Association* in December 2007 revealed that the cost of fruits and vegetables is climbing faster than inflation and that junk food is becoming relatively cheaper.[19] The authors reported that foods with the lowest nutritional value and highest calories were more than ten times less expensive than those with the highest density of nutrients and fewest calories. They suggested that this might be partly why the highest rates of obesity continue to exist in lower-income populations. In chapter 9, we suggest creative remedies for this unfortunate situation, including taxes on junk food and government subsidies for the production and even consumption of healthy, fresh, and whole foods.

The imperative of detoxification
in the face of chemical exposures

Without a healthy planet, it is impossible to have healthy people. Our relationship with Mother Nature is tens of thousands of years old and has proved to be far more complex than we can begin to understand. Intervening unwisely in nature's works is not only arrogant and naïve but also dangerous. We are learning that if we don't take care of our environment, our environment won't take care of us.

It should be a no-brainer that if we put synthetic chemicals into our bodies that are not found in nature, they will likely interfere in some way with the normal metabolism of our cells. We are continually exposed to an estimated 100,000 synthetic chemicals that have been manufactured within the past century or so, and they poison our food, water, air, and soil on a daily basis. In his important book *The Hundred-Year Lie*, mainstream investigative journalist Randall Fitzgerald gives a chilling account of the dire health and environmental consequences of "better living through chemistry" since the introduction of synthetic chemicals early in the 20th century.[20]

These synthetic chemicals frequently interfere with an already stressed cellular metabolism. While most healthy people have the necessary metabolic capacity to compensate to some extent for many of these toxic exposures, sick people very often do not. When we are weakened by illness, some of us decompensate (that is, suffer functional deterioration in a previously working organ or system) from exposure to what may seem trivial to the rest of us. This line of reasoning does not mean that some synthetic chemicals cannot restore and maintain more normal metabolism any more than it means that all chemicals found naturally occurring in nature are good for us. Some pharmaceutical drugs can be lifesaving, but we also know that others can be linked to hundreds of thousands of deaths, whereas only a meager 50 deaths per year or so are caused by natural remedies, herbs, or nutraceuticals.

We are also beginning to appreciate that the residues of many synthetic drugs cause significant damage to our environment in general, posing threats to all living species. The extent of damage to health and to life itself caused by all forms of environmental pollution is probably not even imaginable.

In view of these realities, it is indeed tragic that the concept of detoxification is, as we have noted, greatly underappreciated in mainstream medicine and continues to be largely unaddressed in medical training. Yet it is no more than simple common sense that our bodies cannot function optimally if they have been poisoned by failing internal metabolism or by the accumulation of external toxic exposures.

Studies assessing the extent of toxic-substance accumulation in humans are shocking. Considering that even our polar ice caps are now polluted with a wide range of toxic chemicals, this should not come as a surprise. In a collaborative study jointly conducted by the Environmental Working Group, Commonweal, and Mount Sinai School of Medicine in New York, researchers from two major laboratories found an average of 91 industrial compounds, pollutants, and other chemicals in the blood and urine of nine volunteers, for a total of 167 different toxic chemicals.[21] None of these people worked with chemicals or lived near an industrial facility. The total "body burden" of chemicals in these typical subjects contained the following:

- Seventy-six agents that cause cancer in humans or animals

- Ninety-four that are toxic to the brain and nervous system

- Seventy-nine that cause birth defects or abnormal development in the fetus

Aside from the health challenge that each of these toxins poses, it is troubling that the dangers of exposure to such chemicals *in combination* (known as *chemical synergies*) has never been studied, and many have not been adequately studied individual-ly.[22] According to Randall Fitzgerald, "Chemical synergies may provide an explanation for many of the great mystery illnesses of the late twentieth century—chronic fatigue syndrome, Gulf War syndrome, irritable bowel syndrome, and multiple chemical sensitivity syndrome."[23]

The latter was in fact the malady that my wife, Vicki, suf-fered. Fitzgerald reported that 30 percent of the U.S. population suffers from some symptoms of multiple chemical sensitivity syndrome—double the rate in 1987, according to findings of the National Academy of Sciences that he cites.

The impact of toxic exposures on our health may be more far reaching than anyone has imagined. One dramatic example is cited in a recent article in the *Lancet*, in which the authors spec-ulated that pesticides may play a major role in the epidemic of obesity and Type 2 diabetes that now affects nearly 25 percent of all Americans.[24] They reported a clear association between the levels of *organochlorine pesticides* (a commonly used type of insecticide) in the body and Type 2 diabetes. It may be that these toxic compounds cause inflammation in the body that results in insulin resistance and eventual diabetes, they argue. In *JAMA* in September 2008, British researchers reported an association between a chemical called *bisphenol A* (BPA) and the incidence of both Type 2 diabetes and heart disease.[25] BPA leaches out of poly-carbonate plastic bottles, the coating in most food and beverage cans, and dental sealants.

More dramatic still is our epidemic of cancer. The incidence of almost all types of cancer has gone up an average of 85 percent since 1950, no doubt largely the result of increased toxic expo-sures. From a likelihood of one in three in 1994, the chance that each of us may suffer from cancer in our lifetime is now one in two, stated Fitzgerald.

Genetic defects disturb cellular biochemistry

Genetic defects are far more common than you might imagine, and they should not be underestimated. We all have a unique heredity that is literally our genetic fingerprint. If we don't have the right biochemical tools to sustain the complicated bio-chemistry that underlies our genetic profile, we may be at risk for metabolic disorders such as diabetes, cancer, heart disease, hypertension, stroke, many neurological diseases, and many other disorders. Often, genetic defects remain inconsequential until they are challenged by exposure to environmental toxins or some other stressor.

A wide range of potential genetic defects can influence how and whether our bodies can detoxify what gets into them, how our immune systems defend against foreign chemicals and microbes, and whether we are at risk for developing particular diseases. Genetic testing is becoming more available in clinical practice every year, and physicians increasingly use nutritional biochemistry to circumvent genetic biochemical defects that can lead to disease.

We must also take note of new research documenting that our DNA is not as immutable as was once believed; this research shows that it can dramatically change in response to diet, exercise, stress, and much more. We will address this exciting discovery in a later chapter when we report on the effects of lifestyle on prostate-cancer genes.

Our internal pharmacology is regulated by our thoughts and feelings

The last of the four key factors affecting cellular health is our *psychospiritual* state. What we think and feel has profound effects on our biochemistry and physiology; an enormous, growing mass of research documents the ways in which our thoughts and feelings regulate the internal pharmacy of the body through modulation of the secretion of hormones, endorphins, neurotransmitters, and growth factors, as well their effect on energy production, blood flow, and much more. In return, these factors regulate key physiological functions such as cardiac output, respiration, immunity, digestion, urinary function, detoxification, and even our mood. Numerous authors have noted these body-mind-spirit linkages, including Deepak Chopra, Candace Pert, Beverly Rubik, and Larry Dossey; we cover their findings in more detail in later chapters.

Every individual cell has a highly complex relationship with all the other cells of our body that involves tens of thousands of chemical reactions every millisecond of our lives. These constant changes occur in an incredibly intricate but organized way that keeps our bodies functioning perfectly unless we interrupt the normal process. We understand only a minuscule portion of these amazing relationships between the physical, biochemical, bioenergetic, emotional, and spiritual aspects of who we are. Thank goodness our bodies have the innate ability to simultaneously manage all these amazing factors that keep us functioning and active every moment of our lives—that is, as long as we don't disturb them with destructive thoughts.

Modern medicine is at war with nature

With this brief background on the emerging paradigm of medical science—a key facet of which is based on the factors that affect cellular metabolism—let's return to the competing worldview for a contrasting look.

We've noted that the old approach to medical science is in part modeled on the metaphor of war. Its goal is to defeat illness at almost any cost, acting from a position outside the human body. This war accelerated immensely with the discovery of the germ, which was believed to be responsible for causing disease by invading our bodies. And we have remained at war with these microbes ever since Pasteur's landmark discoveries. Even after the discovery and introduction of antibiotics into medical practice to kill these microscopic invaders, we have persisted in this ongoing fight against nature. In fact, the war escalates every day, and so do the consequences.

For its part, nature has responded to every new antibiotic by developing novel adaptations that create antibiotic-resistant strains of microbes. This has led to the emergence of the lethal bacterium known as *methicillin-resistant staphylococcus aureus* (MRSA), plus several other highly resistant bacteria such as the *pseudomonas* and *C. difficile* pathogens. Even the once-easy-to-treat pneumococcal bacteria have become resistant to many antibiotics. Some microbes are now resistant to *all* man-made antibiotics.

Despite all this, few would argue that the discovery of antibiotics did not make a tremendous difference in fighting infection and saving lives. Yet we can see that this advancement has come at a huge price: Our war against nature has catalyzed a warlike response from nature.

Meanwhile, what about the other end of the Pasteur–Beauchamp spectrum? Why haven't we fully addressed the obvious fact that these opportunistic infections usually attack us when our immunity is depressed? Instead we pursue pharmaceutical and other strategies that are akin to scorched-earth warfare—engaging in battles that both destroy the "enemy" and cause collateral damage to innocent "civilians"—while ignoring the possibility of creating the conditions of well-being in the first place through trade, cultural exchange, negotiation, and conflict resolution.

It has taken more than 50 years to appreciate some of the potentially lethal hazards of using increasingly powerful medicines in isolation from other more natural and supportive strategies. Although we have long known about the microecosystems that inhabit our skin and parts of our respiratory, digestive, and genitourinary systems, we have only recently come to appreciate the significance of interfering with the balances within these systems when we introduce antibiotics into our bodies. These balances are vital to maintaining good health and are profoundly disturbed by antibiotics and a multitude of other factors such as poor diet, stress, immune dysfunction, lack of sleep, poor digestion, a wide variety of pharmaceutical drugs, and numerous miscellaneous factors.

We have come to realize that whenever an antibiotic is introduced to kill a certain microbe that has caused an infection, only those microbes that are able to survive in the presence of the antibiotic will be able to remain in the body; the others, of course, will succumb to the treatment. These ecosystems will remain radically altered until each individual milieu can be restored. This is done by recreating the delicate and sometimes tenuous balance between the defense systems of our bodies and those of the resistant microbes that still reside in the intestinal tract, skin, vagina, tears, and upper-respiratory tract.

Of course, if the bacteria causing a disease are *not* killed by the antibiotic, they can be considered to be especially resilient and may have the potential to become drug-resistant super-strains. It should be remembered that these bugs live in everyone, but they become pathogenic only when their numbers increase above a certain level. When we open up the biological terrain by killing the friendly microbes that protect us, these bacteria overgrow and reach the critical mass they need to cause damage to our tissues.

Because of our inattention to these large issues, MRSA infections are now responsible for thousands of deaths every year in our hospitals. An article published in the *Lancet* in June 2006 reported that more than two million people worldwide now passively carry MRSA in their bodies; MRSA has become part of our new "normal" microflora.[26] These microbes are harmless to most carriers because they persist in only very small numbers. But when they are passed to immunocompromised people—or to those whose use of antibiotics has widened the turf for growth in the gut—the possibility of overgrowth and lethal infection increases dramatically, not only in our hospitals but also out in our communities.

The statistics tell the story: According to an article published in *e-Medicine* in January 2009, 5 percent of all acute-care admissions studied between 1986 and 1998 were complicated by hospital-acquired infections. This amounted to two million infections and 90,000 deaths, at a cost of $4.5 billion annually.[27]

The failure of our war against diseases

The so-called "War on Cancer" that began in the 1970s during President Nixon's era. Despite more than 35 years and hundreds of billions of dollars spent on medical research to conquer cancer, for the most part this war has been a dismal failure. While some claim we've made tremendous strides in treating certain cancers, this malady remains the second leading cause of death in the United States, continuing to kill more than half a million people annually, and will afflict up to 50 percent of us at some time, a far larger percentage than at the outset of this "war." If this is an example of success, I tremble when imagining what the toll might be if it were a failure.

We are also fighting a losing war against Type 2 diabetes. More than 25 percent of all Americans now have the earliest form of Type 2 diabetes, also called *metabolic syndrome*, that can eventually lead to full-blown Type 2 diabetes. Solid data supports the position that Type 2 diabetes is caused by poor diet, lack of exercise, overweight, insufficient sleep, too much stress, toxic environmental exposures, and, to some extent, genetic factors that we have generally falsely assumed to be the major reason we develop diabetes.

Until the diagnosis of metabolic syndrome is made, however, conventional medicine offers almost nothing to proactively reverse its risk factors. The vast majority of research dollars invested in this problem are directed to developing drugs to treat the disease *only after* it has already affected us. What is needed is a widespread prevention program that teaches about a healthy diet, exercise, stress reduction, adequate sleep, and realistic weight management—in other words, an urgent application of the preventive component of the integral-health medicine model, as detailed in chapter 9.

We are also at war against arteriosclerosis, which causes heart attacks, strokes, kidney disease, dementia, and peripheral vascular disease. Have you ever thought of how the term *heart attack* was coined? The word *attack* implies that a war is being fought and the heart is under attack from some outside enemy. This is another example of Pogo's famous statement, "We have met the enemy, and he is us!" Once again, we know that our chances of developing arteriosclerosis of the heart are related to lifestyle issues as well as to such factors as cholesterol and its subfractions—that is, HDL and LDL cholesterol—or to other independent biochemical risk factors such as homocysteine, apolipoproteins, fasting insulin, many coagulation factors, and iron levels. In fact, lifestyle, stress, social, and environmental factors are by far the most important factors. Remember that a hundred years ago, we had pretty much the same genetic makeup. Heart attacks were so rare in those days that they were a medical curiosity!

The complicated high-tech approach that underlies modern medicine's quest to triumph over nature ascribes a God-like quality to medical practitioners and researchers. This belief system has tended to erode the collaboration and partnership between physician and patient—and of the two of them with nature—and has led to the attitude of "We can take care of you, even if you don't take care of yourself" and "You can leave the treatment to us." We have become comfortable relying on an incomplete model of science and medicine to solve our health issues and have relinquished much of our personal responsibility to live a healthy lifestyle and build an ecologically sustainable world. A vast industry—sometimes known as the *medical-pharmaceutical-industrial complex*—has grown around this one-sided model of health care, with its questionable claim of being based upon genuine science.

Let us now examine how well it is serving us.

Four

How Well Is America's Health Care System Working?

*Introducing businesslike practices, the theory went, would
streamline health care and contain costs. But defying the
collective wisdom of America's business schools, just the opposite
happened: A massive bureaucracy has grown up to administer
an ever-larger share of health care dollars in a paperwork factory
that would be the dream of a 1950s Soviet bureaucrat.*

—Donald Bartlett and James Steele, *Critical Condition*

*The performance we get for what we invest in health care is
probably the biggest business failure in American history.*

—*BusinessWeek*, August 26, 2002

We've already alluded to another sad statistic: The United
States does not even rate among the top 30 countries in
the world in terms of overall quality of health care, according to
a ranking by country done by the World Health Organization
(WHO).[1] We are 37th, just after the great modern countries of
Morocco and Costa Rica. America spends hundreds of billions

annually on health care, generates much of the most advanced biomedical research and technology, and attracts the finest minds into its practice of medicine, yet we are not ranked anywhere near the top as a nation. This is simply shocking.

These WHO statistics were reported on the World Health Organization website in June 2000 and represent the last time such a global study has been published. The study measured five elements: life expectancies, inequalities in health, the responsiveness of the system in providing diagnosis and treatment, inequalities in responsiveness, and how fairly systems are financed. Unfortunately, none of these areas have seen improvement in the U.S. since the year 2000.

Our dismal rating is a harsh pill for Americans to swallow—especially given that we also spend far more per capita than any of these countries just to get our mediocre quality of care. In fact, no country spends even half of what we do per person, and yet three dozen have better health care outcomes.

The WHO researchers found, for example, that Americans spent more per person (about $6,000 at that time), yet ranked far below Great Britain, which spent about $2,500 per capita but whose citizens have a greater life expectancy than Americans.

France was rated first in the world in the study. Its health statistics as of 2007 tell much of the story, according to a July 2007 *BusinessWeek* article that praised its system: "France's infant death rate is 3.9 per 1,000 live births, compared with 7 in the U.S., and average life expectancy is 79.4 years, two years more than in the U.S. The country has far more hospital beds and doctors per capita than America, and far lower rates of death from diabetes and heart disease. The difference in deaths from respiratory disease, an often preventable form of mortality, is particularly striking: 31.2 per 100,000 people in France, vs. 61.5 per 100,000 in the U.S."[2]

One piece of embarrassing data in the WHO study indicated that the U.S. was handily beaten by Oman, a tiny oil-rich country on the Arabian Peninsula. The Omanis must be doing something right: They spent less than $350 per person per year in 2000 and yet were ranked in the top ten in the world. Japan, whose lifestyle and economy are more comparable to ours, kept its costs to about one-third of U.S. costs but still ranked in the WHO's top ten. What in the world accounts for such discrepancies?

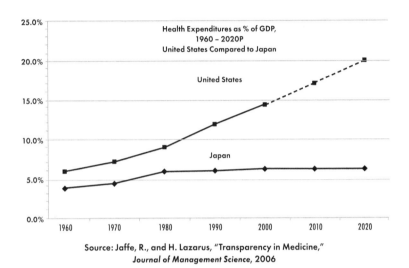

Source: Jaffe, R., and H. Lazarus, "Transparency in Medicine,"
Journal of Management Science, 2006

Figure 4.1. The percentage of gross domestic product spent on conventional health care in the United States compared with that of Japan, 1960–2020.

Our increased spending correlates with a chronic-disease epidemic

So, how did the United States get to be 37th in the world, just one notch above Slovenia? Right after World War II, most aspects of medicine were either run on a nonprofit basis or operated by physicians who saw themselves as professionals, not businesspeople. In those days, low-cost health insurance was available to virtually everyone, including people with existing medical problems; doctors had the time to understand your problems and know you personally, and even make house calls. A hospital stay required only a few days' pay, rather than many months of income. Charity hospitals were available to take care of families that couldn't afford the low-cost hospitals. Regular hospitals rarely had a primary goal of maximizing income; since most were owned by voluntary boards of trustees, church-related groups, or the government, they were simply expected to serve the medical needs of the community. In his helpful book on the subject of the commercialization of the health care industry, *A Second Opinion*, Arnold Relman, MD, of Harvard Medical School explains that, as late as the 1950s, "Few people thought of health care as a market for investment. . . . It was not only an insignificant part of the national economy; it was not even considered to be a commercial enterprise."[3]

But since the 1960s, America has been in a rush to commercialize medicine. Doctors have had to turn into business entrepreneurs rather than pursue the role of compassionate healers; community hospitals that were once nonprofit have become publicly traded, profit-driven national chains; and hundreds of private insurance companies have arisen, competing with each other to make money on actuarial bets against each American's ability to maintain health.

What have been the fruits of all of this "market discipline"?

Contrary to what free-market theory would predict, the data on the ground shows that if the objective is genuine health care, market competition and the profit imperative operate in an *inverse* relationship to what we actually want to achieve. What an irony! We all aspire to maximize the social goods of health, healing, wellness, and longevity; instead, we find that the marketing of disease care correlates with a measurable deterioration in the health status of Americans.

Simply stated, *less* disease care is *better* disease care (provided that it is equitably distributed in the first place) in a rational health care system.

But to the marketers of disease care products and services, more disease—and especially more costly, chronic diseases—*that* is where the money is.

"The very core principle of the market system, that companies will compete by selling more products to everyone, is actually the last thing the health-care system needs," wrote Pulitzer Prize–winning journalists Donald Bartlett and James Steele (who are quoted at the top of this chapter) in their essential book, *Critical Condition*.[4] "The goal should be to sell less, not more—that is, fewer doctor visits, fewer diagnostic tests, fewer hospitalizations, fewer consultations with specialists, and fewer prescription drugs." But try telling *that* to the marketing departments of our leading health care providers!

Consider this bar chart, which dates back to the beginning of the early period of the corporatization of health care:

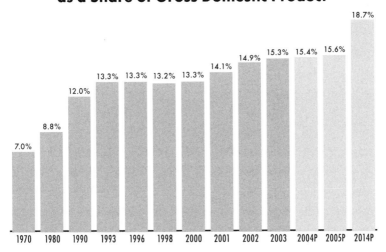

National Health Spending as a Share of Gross Domestic Product

Figure 4.2. The cost of health care as a percentage of America's GDP has more than doubled since 1970. It is now the largest sector of our economy. (Source: Centers for Medicare and Medicaid Services.)

This chart, compiled by the Centers for Medicare and Medicaid Services, clearly shows the extent of our "misspending" on health care as a percentage of gross domestic product (GDP). Starting at about 7 percent in 1970, the percentage had nearly doubled by 2000. It was 16 percent in 2008 and is at 18 percent at the time of writing in early 2009, almost matching the chart's projection for 2015. At the 2009 rate, it should top *20 percent* by 2014, a nearly threefold increase in less than 50 years.

One might argue that these soaring expenditures on sickness care at least contribute to the economy. But why are we getting so much sicker as we spend so much more money? Consider this quick summary of the incidence of chronic disease in the last 50 years, pulled together from a variety of sources:

1. Despite vast expenditures, the cancer rate (which is now approaching one of every two Americans) has seen little or no improvement.

2. Obesity has increased fourfold overall and has tripled to 17 percent in children.

3. Diabetes has increased sixfold—a true epidemic.

4. Heart disease is down but remains officially our number one killer.

5. Medicine itself may be (unofficially) today's leading cause of death.

What has happened to us? Nearly every family in America now has a member with a chronic disease. A prime example is obesity. The prevalence of obesity in the U.S. roughly doubled between 1991 and 2001 in all categories, to about 20 percent of the population, according to the Centers for Disease Control. And in 2008, approximately 127 million adults in the U.S. were overweight, 60 million were obese, and 9 million were extremely obese. This means that about two-thirds of all U.S. adults are overweight, and nearly a third are obese.[5] This is alarming, for obesity has moved into second place as the leading cause of preventable death in the United States. It is significantly associated with diabetes, high blood pressure, asthma, arthritis, and generally poor health.

Just how counterproductive is mainstream medicine?

The rise in our spending on disease care correlates with an increase in the incidence of disease over many decades; of this there can be no doubt. And this strange phenomenon will persist as long as we ignore such things as prevention, public health education, single-payer insurance, and the other reforms recommended later in the book—especially the cost-benefit ratio provided by integrative care with its more practical methodology of treatment. Compounding the irony are what might be called the secondary effects of mainstream medicine; because of their invasive nature, too many mainstream treatments are literally counterproductive.

Studies published by researcher Jason Lazarou et al. in *JAMA* in 1998 estimated that there are over two million adverse drug reactions in hospitals and more than 100,000 in-hospital deaths in the U.S. every year that are attributable to the *expected* "side effects" of pharmaceutical drugs.[6] This number is likely to be higher today. Lazarou's projection does *not* include deaths from the expected side effects of pharmaceutical drugs used on patients outside the hospital. This could become an even more frightening statistic! It also does not include the *mistakes and misuses* of pharmaceutical drugs. This number is difficult to predict, but one would expect it to be substantially higher.

Medical mistakes, known as *iatrogenic* errors, account for another enormous number of deaths. The Institute of Medicine in Washington, DC, estimates 98,000 such deaths each year. However, Dr. Lucian L. Leape's December 1994 article in *JAMA* titled "Error in Medicine" cited some remarkable statistics:

- As far back as 1964, a previous researcher, Schimmel, reported that 20 percent of hospital patients suffered iatrogenic injury, with a 20 percent fatality rate.

- In 1981, Steel reported that 36 percent of hospitalized patients experienced iatrogenesis, with a 25 percent fatality rate, and adverse drug reactions were involved in 50 percent of those injuries.

- In 1991, Bedell reported that 64 percent of acute heart attacks in one hospital were preventable and were mostly due to adverse drug reactions.[7]

Leape went on to point out that the *Harvard Medical Practice Study* published in 1991, using a very conservative 4 percent iatrogenic injury rate for patients and a 14 percent fatality rate on data reported in 1984 from the state of New York, would allow one to project that 180,000 Americans would die each year at least in part as a result of iatrogenic injury. Had he chosen to use the higher percentage rates mentioned in the list above, this number could be increased to well over a million deaths. Such statistics sound more like the outcome of a global war than the benevolent efforts of a health care system.

A much more detailed exposé of the dangers of mainstream medicine is presented in *Death by Medicine*, a controversial research study published in 2003 by natural medicine crusader Gary Null et al.[8] This much-quoted study claims that, based on data from different peer-reviewed journal articles, 783,000 to 999,936 deaths are caused annually by the medical profession, at a cost of $282 billion to $468 billion. In the abstract of the piece, the authors wrote: "A definitive review and close reading of medical peer-review journals and government health statistics shows that American medicine frequently causes more harm than good." If they are correct in their analysis, the American medical system is itself the leading cause of death and injury in the U.S. By comparison, in 2007 the Centers for Disease Control

(CDC) reported that 652,091 Americans died of heart disease and 559,312 died of cancer.

Null's study also found that the annual number of people having in-hospital, adverse drug reactions (ADR) to prescribed medicine was 2.2 million. In 1995, the CDC's Richard Besser, MD, said the annual number of unnecessary antibiotics prescribed for viral infections was 20 million. Besser also reported that by 2003, tens of millions of unnecessary antibiotics prescriptions were written, that 7.5 million unnecessary medical and surgical procedures were performed, and that the number of people exposed to unnecessary hospitalization annually was 8.9 million.[9, 10, 11, 12]

Some have disputed these conclusions, pointing out that the authors did not factor in how many lives are *saved* by modern medicine annually or consider the incidence of other *positive* effects that result in increased quality of life. For example, one set of critics of the study, a group of mainstream physicians, quite appropriately state on their website Science-Based Medicine: "Drug reactions? All effective drugs also have side effects. It's meaningless to count the side effects without counting the benefits. An insulin reaction counts as an adverse drug reaction, but if the patient weren't taking insulin he probably wouldn't be alive to have a reaction. Some of the counted drug reactions are transient minor annoyances like a rash. People have iatrogenic infections in the hospital, for instance post-op infections; but without hospitalization and surgery they might have been dead instead of just being infected. Iatrogenic deaths? How many of those were of people who would have died many years earlier without modern medical care? How many of those iatrogenic causes were high-risk treatments in high-risk patients who had no other option?"[13]

On the other hand, the Null study mightily challenges our assumptions about the status quo in medicine. True, thousands of medical journal articles provide fragmentary data showing that the quality of life and life extension are the direct effects of some mainstream medical strategies. Yet there is no data showing an overall net benefit from the effects of medical practice—neither in increasing overall longevity nor in saving lives. And the numbers that Null has cited show, without a doubt, that the *cost–benefit ratio* of mainstream health care in America is poor in the extreme. Adding even more irony, there is some data documenting that when hospital physicians have gone on strike, mortality rates have decreased!

Given its posture of a war on nature, it is evident that modern medicine takes far too many risks for too much money. The obvious antidote is to adopt what may be called *a hierarchy of treatment modalities.* The methodology of integral-health medicine as I now practice it requires—for the sake of safety, effectiveness, and cost—that the least invasive therapy should be utilized first in all cases. Generally, the order of consideration should be as follows:

- Lifestyle strategies such as a healthy diet, adequate sleep and exercise, stress reduction, weight control, avoidance of toxic exposures, and securing emotional and spiritual balance in life are the *first line of defense.*

- Noninvasive complementary and alternative (CAM) services such as acupuncture, herbal medicine, chiropractic, bodywork, homeopathy, and energy medicine are *the next line of defense.*

- Natural-medicine approaches based on the latest advances in orthomolecular medicine, functional medicine, and bioenergetic research—and inclusive of advanced forms of testing—are a *further line of defense.*

- Very careful and sparing use of pharmaceutical drugs, surgery, and other invasive strategies are *the last line of defense.*

What would it take to orient today's medicine according to this simple and reasonable protocol? As they say, dear reader, follow the money.

A health care system at the breaking point

It is increasingly evident that without radical reform of our health care system, we will have a system that not only delivers relatively poor health, but also cripples our national economy and federal budget.

We've reached the limit of how much can be spent before we begin to witness failures in various sectors of global business by American companies. The most salient example of the magnitude of this problem is our ailing automotive industry. General Motors (GM), for example, spent a staggering $4.8 billion on health care in 2006, more than it spent on steel for building cars that year. At the time, many people joked that GM was actually a giant health insurance provider that happens to make cars. By comparison, foreign competitors to GM operate in countries that have comprehensive national health insurance, so they face a very minor burden. This is one reason why Japanese brands were thriving just as GM was approaching bankruptcy in 2008 before it had to be bailed out by the federal government. "These days," wrote the *New York Times* on May 19, 2006, "health care costs are causing enormous financial headaches for the Big Three. GM has an unfunded liability of $85 billion in today's money to cover future health care costs for workers and retirees. That is seven to eight times the market value of the whole company. General Motors estimates that health care costs add about $1,500 to the cost of each vehicle it makes in the United States. Chrysler claims a health care cost of $1,400 per vehicle. Ford says its burden is $1,100. . . . Japanese companies face little of this burden in Japan, where the government covers retirees' health care and pays a bigger share of workers' pensions."[14]

Numbers just like these can be found all across major American industries that compete internationally. No wonder our major corporations are beginning to favor comprehensive reform in the way we finance health care. A clear-headed businessperson in possession of the facts, and who is not encumbered by Washington politics, can easily conclude that we must shift to a genuine health care paradigm with an emphasis on prevention, objective science, and integrative care, concurrently with a move toward national insurance for all workers and citizens. Such an insight gives new meaning to the old statement that, "What's good for GM is good for America."

Let's look at some more numbers: Health care spending rose to $2.4 trillion in 2008, a 9 percent increase over $2.2 trillion in 2007, according to the Centers for Medicare and Medicaid Services. This was more than double the rise in GDP that year, which was 3.5 percent in 2008.

We've earlier noted that we easily spend twice as much per person as any other industrialized country, even though we slid to last place among these same countries in preventing deaths through timely and effective medical care.

The 2005 report of the Boards of Trustees for Medicare given annually to the Congress estimated that providing promised Medicare benefits over just the next ten years could require nearly $3 trillion in new tax revenues; but raising taxes by that amount, it said, would eliminate over 800,000 jobs in each of those years.

We've noted the correlation of higher costs with more disease. What then are the factors *causing* these excessive rates of inflation?

According to a widely noted article in the September 2000 issue of *Archives of Internal Medicine,* our unsustainable health care costs are directly related to excessive administrative services resulting from a fragmented system, escalating malpractice insurance costs passed through to patients, uncontrolled use of expensive technologies, overtreatment at the end of life, lack of continuity of care, and excessive pharmaceutical drug use, among the leading causes. Yet, the authors claim, "the number of Americans with optimal health care has diminished such that they have become an 'endangered species.'"[15]

Our own analysis pins the problem not only on a disconnected litany of issues, but even more so on the system that underlies and produces each one: We lay in wait for symptoms to appear, and then focus on overkill treatments, and blend this approach with an irrational system of health insurance.

The proper charter of any for-profit health insurer is to maximize profit for shareholders—that part is "rational." The best strategy for achieving this goal is to skim off, from the top of the pool of the entire population, only the healthiest customers—while leaving the rest of the population largely dependent on government or emergency services. Of course, the net social effect of this line of attack is irrational. It drives up costs because the poor or those with preexisting conditions lack access to prevention, education, and affordable routine care, forcing them to enter the system *only* when they have no choice but to resort to expensive acute care.

Structurally, our private health insurance system consists of hundreds of competing providers. Each one sells to a highly fragmented universe of purchasers of health plans—ranging from institutional buyers such as General Motors, to businesses of all kinds, and to ordinary citizens or families. Of course, such a fractured pool of purchasers puts all buyers not eligible for Medicare or Medicaid at a large disadvantage. Americans buying private insurance have far less power to negotiate for lower prices, compared with single-payer systems such as that in Canada, which buy on behalf of the entire population.

Aside from its negotiating advantage, each private insurer incurs higher costs—which it must pass on as higher premiums—to cover the cost of marketing to this splintered pool against numerous competitors. Other costs unique to this system include the expense of sifting out the less risky customers that are more profitable to cover, and dealing with billing disputes from doctors.

We pay two to three times more than other countries for health services—says former senator Tom Daschle, a leading health care policy expert—because of "the complexity, marketing costs, and insurance overhead that result from our market-oriented system," including 31 percent alone for administrative overhead—compared, for example, with 17 percent for Canada. Amazingly, America's doctors and nurses, he says, "spend between one-third and one-half of their time completing paperwork."[16]

In the final analysis, our commercialized health care system, including the way that insurance is managed, supports and profits from the assumption that virtually all health problems should be reduced to medical diagnoses of disease symptoms that are managed with prescription drugs or other high-tech solutions. This system's potential for the greatest profit lies in treating symptoms and dealing with acute crises or chronic conditions, and in seeing the costs and volume of this sort of business increase indefinitely. Can you see why, politically and in terms of profitability, the disease care system favors treatment of symptoms over curing or healing, after-the-fact care for acute illness over prevention, expensive drugs over simple nutrients and herbs, and a fragmented private insurance system over a national single-payer solution?

Hospitals, HMOs, and the central role of the insurance industry

Not *everything* in our current system militates against cost control. Given the spiraling inflation generated by the disease care system, it is no wonder that we've witnessed the emergence of cost-oriented managed care companies that are pressuring physicians to treat diseases as cheaply as possible within the disease care approach—if for nothing else, to leave room for their own profits. In this mentality, time is money, and this reality, coupled with the burgeoning cost of high-tech medicine, makes it difficult to justify paying for more than the bare minimum of expenses required to get people on their feet. To enforce this approach, many key health care decisions are no longer in the hands of highly trained physicians, as they were up until the last few decades; today, private insurance companies, HMOs (health maintenance organizations), or for-profit hospitals call the shots.

In most respects, insurance companies prevail. For example, as costs throughout the system have continued to soar out of control, insurers have found it necessary to dictate who gets hospitalized and for how long; thus, many conditions are now treated on an outpatient basis when years ago the patients would have been admitted to be on the safe side. To stay in business, hospitals must follow binding contractual agreements that have clear restrictions preventing hospitalization for certain conditions. Hours are often wasted on the phone in an effort to obtain permission from insurance companies to admit certain borderline cases. If patients are admitted but coverage is denied, the hospitals have to eat those losses themselves.

Hospital administrators are often thrust into an unfair position. Not only might they have to deny coverage to many people whom they know deserve more treatment than they are getting, but also they must explain this to the physicians and nurses who have to tell patients and their families that they cannot help them. Some of these situations lead to medical disasters, even resulting in lawsuits for malpractice.

It is not hard to imagine how difficult it must be for some physicians to deny certain patients admission to the hospital when they know that it is neither wise nor safe to send the patients back home for care. Doctors are often caught on the horns of a dilemma: While it is surely tough to say no to patients for some services, if physicians take matters into their own hands and override hospital policy, they must then answer to their employer. In many instances, physicians who have cared enough to jeopardize their jobs have been fired.

No wonder that the business contingent of our health care system is the only sector that seems to be happy with the present state of affairs. And why shouldn't they be happy? They've achieved what they set out to accomplish—bringing "marketplace values" to health care—and they've made serious money in the process. They promised to make health care a profitable business enterprise, and to "do what they could" for patients. They have largely succeeded in their mission.

One of the key objectives of commercialized health care was—for the sake of "efficiency"—to remove the independence of physicians. At the beginning of this process in the 1980s, many holdouts were determined to continue practicing in the style they believed patients deserved and good medicine required; they simply could not imagine practicing medicine HMO style. They would not sell out their patients to HMO conglomerates, simply because it was the wrong thing to do. But by the early 1990s, the already intense pressure on physicians to join HMOs had escalated to the point where it became almost impossible to escape their tentacles. Even the most well-intentioned physicians could not stand up to the severe economic pressure exerted by the lower prices for service and insurance offered by HMOs to individuals and organizations. As a result, doctors with independent practices simply crumbled. Yet for me, it was still a shock to witness the buyout of one medical practice after the next by the giant medical insurance industry, hospitals, and independent physician organizations.

Physicians are discontented with today's medical practice

As a result of this history, the discontent with America's health care system is widespread among physicians. You would know this for a fact if—like me—you were within earshot of daily conversations among physicians. I can assure you that the same set of complaints I routinely hear is being aired in thousands of doctors' hospital lounges throughout the country.

I can also testify to the fact that the nature of these conversations has dramatically changed over the past 30 years. Physicians used to spend most of their time sharing stories about patients' problems, looking for the best solutions for difficult situations, and socializing. This nurturing camaraderie kept spirits high.

Physicians experienced the satisfaction of working together to help their patients; there was great pride in being a physician on the frontlines of assisting patients on their way back to health. We also experienced a sense of intellectual freedom: Within wide guidelines, the type of medical practice applied was up to each individual physician. For the most part, there was no one to answer to other than patients, their families, and one's conscience.

But today's physicians have essentially become employees of large business conglomerates. Often there's not much they can do to influence how their patients are treated. The human element—the caring and healing, the attention to family needs, and the focus on service—has taken a back seat to profitability. While doctors still share with each other stories of interesting and difficult-to-manage patients, the hottest topics in doctors' lounges are now related to the increased volume of work, procedural administrative obstacles that must be hurdled before even beginning to address solving patient problems, the impracticality of finding sufficient time to help patients, and, of course, their ever-growing financial challenges. For many physicians, this state of affairs has led to utter discontent, frustration, and at times outright anger.

Compared with the good old days, an atmosphere of gloom and despair has descended. Sadly, many highly skilled and valued physicians have left their practices. They are "retiring early." Only a few have been able to maintain a private practice and continue treating patients the way they used to—the way that they know in their hearts is the right way. Consequently, not only is there a growing shortage of physicians, but also we are losing some of our most treasured healers.

Several surveys measuring physician satisfaction with conventional medicine have produced shocking results. A 2002 Kaiser Family Foundation Survey of 2,608 physicians disclosed that over a five-year period, 60 percent had a decrease in enthusiasm toward their medical practice, 87 percent believed that physician morale had decreased, and 75 percent felt that managed care had had a negative impact on how they were practicing medicine. The reasons for their displeasure included the following:

- Too much paperwork (74 percent)
- Not enough time for their families, hobbies, or friends (56 percent)
- Dissatisfaction with their lack of autonomy (54 percent)[17]

In a study of 4,500 women physicians regarding career satisfaction that was published in *Archives of Internal Medicine* in 1999, 31 percent stated that they would not choose to be a physician again, and 38 percent said they would prefer to change their specialty.[18] Physicians such as Rachel Naomi Remen and Lee Lipsenthal now offer classes to help their fellow physicians avoid job burnout by addressing the subject of finding balance in their lives—courses for "healing the healer."

Physicians as well have human needs

Physicians continue to be a special breed of human being committed to serving humanity. At the same time, is important to remember that they have human needs and are vulnerable to the value system of our culture, just like the rest of us. Their apparent decision to put the financial security of their families before the welfare of their patients may seem unfair or wrongheaded, but it is what happened. And it is understandable.

Yet this was not a decision made with a great deal of foresight. Today, physicians are paying dearly for this poor choice made under duress. Sadly, the panic accompanying the threats implied by the giant HMOs scared them to either join or face the possibility of being financially squeezed out of clinical practice entirely. They became convinced that they had to choose between doing the right thing—staying in practice to provide quality, personalized care—or risk losing their patients to the lower-cost managed care providers. The choice amounted to almost certain financial ruin—or joining the massive exodus from private clinical practice into HMO medicine and hoping for the best. I believe that most of them now wish they had done something collectively to prevent the catastrophe that has resulted.

What would you do if you had to make this choice? Had they been loyal to their patients rather than to HMOs, their ability to support their families in the style they had become accustomed to would have been compromised. The system was simply too big and too powerful for all but a few to seriously consider resisting.

As the transition from private practice to medicine driven by private insurance and HMOs deepened, it became relatively easy for large business conglomerates to bribe physicians with what appeared to be handsome prices to purchase their practices. It seemed too risky to go it alone and too easy to give in when they were guaranteed jobs for several years, where there would be plenty of patients and substantial up-front cash settlements to purchase their practices.

The acute problems of private health insurance

We all know that Medicare provides coverage for all citizens over 65, Medicaid covers the poorest of the poor and the disabled, and the Veterans Administration covers all the health care needs of our veterans. Let's look more closely at everyone else. Because of skyrocketing costs for medical care as well as other systemic problems, far too many Americans who do not fall within these three categories simply do not have health insurance. More than 47 million *working* Americans don't have access to health care, or about 16 percent of the population—up from 12 percent in 1980. This large sector of America represents the "working poor." They make too much to qualify for Medicaid but too little to pay for private health insurance—or they work for small businesses that don't offer health insurance.

In addition, roughly 100 million are underinsured. As we learned from the outrageous stories narrated in Michael Moore's provocative film *Sicko*, Americans may have some sort of insurance, but it very often does not come close to covering the costs they may incur if they become sick or injured. It is almost never enough when a major illness strikes. We all know, of course, that the Byzantine, wasteful, and yet highly profitable insurance industry writes all sorts of restrictions into its policies. These loopholes, caps, and exclusions guarantee that most of the underinsured are vulnerable to disaster.

It may not be surprising to learn that the probability of being uninsured depends in part on one's race and where one lives. In 1997, *USA Today* reported that the percentage of uninsured people varied from a low of 8 percent in Wisconsin to 24 percent in Arizona. The percentage of uninsured was 34 for Hispanics, 22 for African-Americans, and only 11 for Caucasians. According to the U.S. Census Bureau, in 2007 these numbers improved very slightly to 32 percent for Hispanics, 19.5 percent for African-Americans, and 11 percent for Caucasians.

According to a study published by the Commonwealth Fund in 2007, the five top-ranked states for affordable health insurance were Hawaii, Iowa, New Hampshire, Vermont, and Maine. The five worst-performing states were Oklahoma, Mississippi, Texas, Arkansas, and Nevada. An article in the August 28, 2008, issue of the *Boston Globe* ranked Massachusetts first overall among states in the proportion of residents with health coverage, with only 7.9 percent not covered, and a report in the August 27, 2008, issue of the *New York Times* ranked Texas last among states, with 24.4 percent of residents having no health coverage. Where you live in the United States obviously matters.

Further, if all states reached the levels of the top ranked, the Commonwealth Fund estimated that 90,000 deaths could be avoided, 22 million people could gain health insurance, and the government's Medicare insurance program could save at least

$22 billion. The report found a strong link between access to health care coverage, particularly insurance, and high-quality care.

According to the *Kaiser/Commonwealth 1997 National Survey of Health Insurance*, the underinsured are four times more likely to defer needed health care or medication than those who have health insurance.[19] This report went on to further document which Americans did get guaranteed health care—congresspeople, the military, qualified veterans, criminals in prisons, Native Americans living on reservations, the indigent, the rich, and those over age 65 who qualified for Medicare.

The Commonwealth Fund's study *Gaps in Health Insurance: An All-American Problem*, completed in January 2006, documented that 41 percent of Americans with an annual income between $20,000 and $40,000 were uninsured for at least part of the previous year. In 2001, this number was only 28 percent.[20] Lower-income families remained the hardest hit, and 67 percent of the underinsured were in families where at least one person was working full-time. They discovered that one in five adults was paying off medical debt, and nearly 60 percent of uninsured adults with chronic illness could not afford their medications. Many of these people ended up in an emergency room or hospital because they didn't have access to a primary care physician. They were also more likely to go without preventive health care services such as screening for cancer, stroke, diabetes, hypertension, and heart disease.

It should be added, of course, that many working Americans who lack employer-provided coverage, would rather not rely on emergency rooms, and earn too much to qualify for Medicaid find themselves forking over the full cost of private insurance. This figure is astronomical if they have preexisting conditions.

The sad consequence of market-driven health care

Hillary Clinton's storied health care reform plan in the early 1990s had the strong potential to solve many of the cost-containment and delivery problems we have outlined. But the largest stakeholders at the time each found aspects that were problematic, leading to its sound rejection. The underlying premise of the thousand-page report that resulted from this courageous effort was to provide *universal health coverage* for all Americans. The bulk of the coverage was to be paid for by employers through payroll taxes and was to be delivered through "carefully regulated" competition between large nonprofit health maintenance organizations such as the Kaiser Plan and Blue Cross, or by the for-profit pre-paid plans that were springing up across the country. The government would cover the cost of membership in a health maintenance organization for the unemployed. The plan also proposed creating "regional alliances" of health care providers who would be subject to a fee-for-service schedule. And states would receive federal funding to administer the program.

Upon the failure of Hillary Clinton's initiative, health policy leaders across the country became convinced that by setting up a competitive marketplace, for-profit managed care organizations and other major care organizations could solve our health care–related economic problems. This trend toward "market solutions" was long under way by the end of the 1980s, and it unfolded through a series of steps: First, medical costs were lowered to some extent by reducing hospital stays. Next, providers systematically reduced payments to physicians, physician groups, and hospitals. At the same time, services were reduced by making it difficult to access specialists and expensive tests, treatments, and medications. Finally, managed care organizations lessened their risks by offering *capitated care.* In this setting, each physician or physician group is paid according to how many patients they are willing to assume care for. If a particular group of patients happened to be especially sick, physicians would have to work harder to provide care but would receive no additional compensation. Needless to say, because this was a competitive business, many physicians and physician groups underestimated the costs of providing health care services and were eventually forced out of business.

Physicians became increasingly squeezed, and, as you may have already guessed, the increased profits did not lead to a reduction in health insurance premiums for individuals.

So, if medical costs went down somewhat, who benefited from managed care if it wasn't the patients or the physicians? You guessed right again: Stockholders and HMO executives made billions of dollars. According to the *1995 Crystal Report* on executive compensation, the total incomes and benefits of health care CEOs were staggering. The top incomes were $14 million for Healthsource Inc., $13 million for Foundation Health Corp., and $6 million for United Health Care Corp. And it has gone up from there in subsequent years.

An article published August 23, 2007, by WebMD showed that the growth of CEO salaries of health insurance companies continued to soar, although the tough times that began in late 2008 have lessened the upward pressure somewhat. For example, it reported that the CEO of United Health Group, William McGuire, was paid $124.8 million in 2005 and has a five-year contract for $342 million. The CEO of Cigna, H. Edward Hanway, was paid $13.3 million in 2005 and given a five-year contract for $62.8 million. Larry Glasscock, CEO of WellPoint, earned $23 million in 2005 and was given a five-year contract for $46.8 million.[21]

Medicare may be the prime example of the slaughter of health care services. Its medical expenses in 1999 were actually cut, and many governmental agencies were bragging about the accomplishment. You might ask yourself how this was possible in an era of increasingly expensive technology and treatment, along with a steadily growing population over the age of 65, all of this occurring against the backdrop of an epidemic of chronic diseases. Something didn't add up.

The only way Medicare costs could be held in check was to cut reimbursements to physicians, other health care providers, and hospitals. Unfortunately, when physicians and other health care providers are paid less, they generally feel the need to see more patients in order to continue generating the income they are accustomed to living on. Inevitably, this results in less time for patient visits as well as more mistakes, because there simply isn't enough time to be with patients or weigh important decisions that could lead to serious errors.

This problem is even worse in the hospital setting, where hospital staffs are often cut to reduce costs, so that fewer nurses, technicians, social workers, psychologists, and specialized services are available for patient care. It seems that while we've contained costs to some extent, we've forgotten what it was that we set out to do in the first place, which was to help the sick.

The result is clear: Managed care cut costs by reducing services, and neither consumer nor physician benefited. Physicians have been put into a conflict-of-interest predicament. They are now frequently being rewarded for seeing more patients in less time, making fewer referrals, and spending less money. What would you expect, given that HMO medicine is above all profit driven—and service oriented only when it is not too much of an economic burden?

Ask yourself once again: How could a country that spends more per person on research, pharmaceutical drugs, technology, insurance, and hospitalizations than any other country in the world offer quality of care across all classes of Americans that is not much better than that of Cuba? The only way this could happen would be if delivery of the best health care in the world were not the primary goal. On the other hand, the dire condition of American health care reported in this chapter makes perfect sense if the primary goal is to keep this sector of the economy profitable, while enriching the businesses, financiers, and major stockholders who own or run health care companies.

Five

The Karma of Big Pharma: Questioning the Drug Industry

It's hard not to note the irony: the generation of Americans who rebelliously experimented with drugs is now a generation upon whom drugs are experimented, with barely a squeak of protest. . . . Has managed care, with its stingy allocation of resources for face-to-face medicine, made pills the de facto primary care physician, Dr. Merck, M.D.?

—Greg Critser, *Generation Rx*

E ven in my earliest days as a doctor, I would become aware now and then of the perils of medical fundamentalism— that is, scientific reductionism based on the objectification of nature, detachment from our patients, and a narrow focus on symptoms of the body. But as I developed a thriving practice, I slowly realized how dependent I was on tools derived from this model of medical science—techniques and technologies for diagnosing and treating diseases, and especially pharmaceutical drugs that only temporarily relieved my patients' symptoms, when they worked at all. I was gradually beginning to face the fact that I rarely addressed the underlying causes of my patients' diseases and that many of my patients were not getting much better.

My final departure from the old model came on the heels of my disillusionment with the efficacy and safety of the vast majority of pharmaceuticals. The epiphany I experienced because of my wife's breakthrough some years later, as described in chapter 1, was the culmination of a long process of disenchantment.

But let's be fair about this controversial subject. If we narrow our focus to the domain of acute care, it can't be denied that the pharmaceutical industry has made significant contributions, notably in its ability to reduce pain and suffering through the suppression of symptoms. Plus, we are now on the cusp of making future breakthroughs in a wide range of conditions that have been largely untreatable. All of us await what the future holds in such hot areas of research as stem cells, genetics, light therapies, biotechnology, bioenergetics, and aspects of quantum physics—some of which may result in pharmaceutical treatments.

Yet we can't let the limited achievements of the pharmaceutical industry eclipse our awareness of its many failings, including the evidence of its occasional fraudulent practices and the many times when drugs have caused outright disasters. Given the industry's dismal track record of safety and reliability, it's not just a cute expression to say that "Big Pharma has bad karma."

The $200 billion pharmaceutical sector is possibly the richest industry in the world—with profits rivaled only by those of big oil, at least before the current economic downturn. But what we find when we look closely, by all independent accounts, is an industry that relies on propaganda, political corruption, and outright deception to obscure its downside—that is, the downstream costs it pushes off onto patients, doctors, and governments, to name a few of its victims. Yet, through its many machinations, sales and profits have continued to outpace those in any comparable sector of the economy.

In a word, Americans are not getting better on the whole because of their lavish use of pharmaceuticals; instead, they are becoming *dependent*.

For example, the use of drugs (almost all for chronic diseases) went from seven prescriptions per person annually in 1993 to double that a decade later; by 2004, almost half of all Americans were taking at least one prescription a day, and one in six was taking more than three a day. Use tapered off a bit after the onset of the recession in 2008.[1] How does Pharma achieve this feat? Let's first look at the bizarre commercial phenomenon known as the *direct-to-consumer* (DTC) ads that we now regularly see on TV. These ads are an almost uniquely American approach to drug education; they're banned in all countries worldwide, except for the U.S. and New Zealand.

The impact of direct-to-consumer drug ads

I am distressed to admit that, like most Americans and many of my medical colleagues, I once accepted without much question the worldview that underlies DTC ads. The core intention of DTC commercials is, of course, to entirely bypass the medical profession and appeal directly to consumers, hoping to induce them to ask their doctors for a remedy for some real malady or for a supposed illness newly identified (read: created) by the drugmaker itself; one study estimated that for every minute the average television viewer spends with his physician each year, he is exposed to *100 minutes of DTC ads.*[2]

These ads characteristically exaggerate the benefits of the drugs being marketed and play down their negative side effects. Many Americans still under the spell of our faulty health care paradigm continue to uncritically accept the illusions created by these advertisements, with their surreal litany of side effects quickly recited in the background while in the foreground we watch perfectly lit images of healthy, happy actors living and loving joyously in soap opera settings.

Do DTC ads work? One thorough study showed that patients' requests due to watching drug ads "have a profound effect" on getting physicians to prescribe antidepressants.[3] No wonder the amount spent on DTC ads has increased from $200 million in 1997—when the FDA eased up on its requirement that all details of side effects must be listed—to over $5 billion in 2007.[4] The FDA also eased up in most other ways possible: In the ten-year period from 1997 to 2007, its warning or enforcement letters to drugmakers over deceptive advertising practices went from 140 to only 20, according to Public Citizen's Health Research Group. Plus, a Government Accountability Office (GAO) report released in November 2006 found that the FDA reviews only a small portion of the ads submitted by drugmakers.

Under the onslaught of this promotional bombardment, we don't realize that we're being programmed to feel better about the dangers being reported; they're simply glossed over and accepted as a normal part of the package of modern high-tech medicine. Also skipped over is the often poor or financially compromised "science" behind these "discoveries," their general ineffectiveness, and the financial burden they place on patients. Not to mention more than 100,000 deaths each year, earlier noted, from adverse reactions to drugs *properly* prescribed and taken, in hospitalized patients alone.

Of course, this figure underestimates the potential danger from these toxic substances. Researchers agree that one drug *alone*, Vioxx, which we discussed in chapter 3, caused as many as 100,000 deaths worldwide before it was finally removed from the market. Drugmaker Merck withdrew Vioxx in September 2004, in what *USA Today* called "a stunning denouement for a blockbuster drug that had been marketed in more than 80 countries with worldwide sales totaling $2.5 billion in 2003."[5] Vioxx had been trumpeted in DTC ads by the likes of Olympic gold medalists Dorothy Hamill and Bruce Jenner, and had been sold in the United States for more than five years.

The FDA had noted problems with Vioxx's side effects early on, and in April 2000 the FDA required Merck to add labeling information about a possible link to such problems. Clearly, the warning was ineffective, as two million Americans were taking Vioxx when it was finally pulled. "Critics describe the rise and fall of Vioxx," wrote *USA Today*, "as a cautionary tale of masterful public relations, aggressive marketing and ineffective regulation." In regard to regulatory oversight by the FDA, *USA Today* went on: "Sen. Chuck Grassley, R-Iowa, says the FDA was worse than passive." It turns out that FDA researcher David Graham, lead scientist on a study that linked Vioxx to more than 27,000 heart attacks or sudden cardiac deaths before it was withdrawn, told Grassley's Senate Finance Committee investigators that *the FDA tried to block publication of his findings.* "Dr. Graham described an environment where he was 'ostracized,' 'subjected to veiled threats' and 'intimidation.'"[6]

Another disturbing case among many others of this ilk concerns several drugs used in the treatment of Type 2 diabetes. Two of these drugs, Avandia and Rezulin, work by increasing the body's sensitivity to insulin through interactions with as many as 100 genes. Even though science doesn't yet know what most of these genes do, a "real time" global experiment on millions of people began when these drugs were introduced in the 1990s.

The first to blow up was Rezulin. It was removed from the market in 2000 after 63 people died from acute liver failure and another 40 victims had to have liver transplants.[7]

Avandia also went south but still remains available. An article published in the June 2007 issue of the *New England Journal of Medicine (NEJM)* documented that Avandia raises the risk of heart death by 64 percent and of heart attack by 43 percent.[8] The then-president-elect of the American Diabetes Association and professor at the University of North Carolina, John Buse, MD, wrote a letter to the FDA in March 2000 stating that there was "a worrisome trend in cardiovascular deaths and severe adverse events" among patients using this drug. He went on to accuse the drugmaker of "rampant abuse of clinical trial data." Avandia is still sold by GlaxoSmithKline, annually grossing more than $2 billion.[9]

Behind every big deception is usually a big motive, and Big Pharma certainly has one: In 2002, a peak year for the industry, we find that "the combined profits for the ten drug companies in the Fortune 500 ($35.9 billion) were more than the profits for all the other 490 businesses put together ($33.7 billion)." This is just one of the astounding facts cited by Marcia Angell, MD, in her 2004 book *The Truth About the Drug Companies.* Angell is a former editor of *NEJM* and one of the most prominent critics of the industry. Drug companies at the time also ranked far above all other industries in average net return, sometimes double and triple that of any other sector, she documented.[10]

We are all mere humans whose natural tendency is to focus on any glimmer of hope for quickly ridding ourselves of our pain and our symptoms, without much effort on our part. Drugmakers manipulate this sentiment. And besides, if their drugs were really that dangerous, certainly the FDA would not allow them to be on the market, right? Wrong. According to critics like Angell, the track record shows that the FDA—when it is functional at all—has lent its seal of approval to one lethal drug after another, often allowing them to be marketed even as the death toll rose. Don't forget that two million Americans were taking Vioxx when it was pulled—despite well-known evidence that it caused cardiac arrest and strokes.

The bottom line is that if one were to truly listen to DTC ads and do just a small bit of research into the drugs being touted, few of us in our right minds would consider taking most of these drugs without serious reservations.

Do you still want to take the purple pill?

Studies have shown that physicians have mixed feelings about the effect of DTC ads on their patients; they realize that patients are often confused about both the efficacy and the associated risks of the drugs being advertised.

Of course, we physicians do know, or should know, just how dangerous and often ineffective drugs are; it's a significant part of our training—and more so now than ever. Yet the environment in which we operate leads us to underplay their problems, as did I in my early years of practice. For example, when was the last time your physician took you aside to explain all the possible side effects and contraindications of a drug he or she asked you to take? For that matter, when has your doctor accompanied such a discussion with a presentation of potential *alternatives*, such as healthier lifestyle or CAM options that might include nutraceuticals or other natural remedies that usually have *no* side effects? The typical discussion in today's mainstream clinic is restricted to explaining the benefits of a drug for a few minutes, and almost no time is spent covering harmful side effects. Of course, this serves to maintain patients' illusion that they have just found an effortless shortcut to restoring their health, one with few or no adverse consequences.

One important study from the University of California, San Diego Medical Center documented that physicians have a *low awareness* of drug side effects relative to their patients, who are, of course, the ones actually suffering painful or uncomfortable side effects. Reported in the *Washington Post* in a piece called "Is Your Doctor in Denial?" the study found that the patients' concerns about the side effects they were experiencing from statin drugs were either ignored or dismissed.[11] According to this study, "Patients reported that they and not the doctor most commonly initiated the discussion regarding the possible connection of drug to symptom [i.e., a drug side effect]. Physicians were reportedly more likely to deny than affirm the possibility of a connection. Rejection of a possible connection [by the physician] was reported to occur even for symptoms with strong literature support for a drug connection." These findings led the researchers to conclude that physicians may too often fail to make an "adverse drug event report" to the FDA on the patients' use of statins, which leads to an underestimation of the incidence of many problems with this class of drugs and the assumption that they are far safer than they really are.

Jerry Avorn, associate professor of medicine at Harvard University and the author of *Powerful Medicines: The Benefits, Risks, and Costs of Prescription Drugs* (Knopf, 2004), stated in the same article, "We already know that there is horrendous underreporting of side effects. *Ninety to ninety-nine percent of serious side effects are not reported by doctors* [emphasis added]." The article went on, "Tracking a drug's safety once it hits pharmacies—so-called post-market surveillance—is a critical part of keeping patients safe, particularly since clinical trials with limited enrollees and a limited study period cannot catch every side effect."[12]

Information about the dangers of approved pharmaceutical drugs must, by law, be provided by pharmaceutical companies and is readily available in the peer-reviewed medical literature that is described in detail in *The Physicians' Desk Reference* (*PDR*). This publication is required by the FDA to be made available to physicians. If you ever have the opportunity to look through the *PDR*, you will be impressed with the more than 3,000 pages of very small print on very big pages. The bulk of its pharmaceutical information is devoted to side effects, warnings, precautions, and contraindications. Yet physicians evidently don't pay much attention to what is printed. If they did, it is hard to believe that they would use pharmaceutical drugs nearly as often as they do. Instead, as happened after my awakening, they would be searching for safer and more effective alternatives!

All told, about a fifth of all drugs that gain full FDA approval ultimately either have a *black box warning* (indicating that the drug carries a significant risk of serious or even life-threatening effects) or else will be withdrawn from the market because of such adverse effects. Nonetheless, pharmaceutical drugs remain the major basis for much of today's medical practice armamentarium. This is the case even though "only a handful of truly important drugs have been brought to market in recent years, and they were mostly based on taxpayer-funded research at academic institutions, small bio-technology companies, or the National Institutes of Health (NIH)," wrote former *New England Journal of Medicine* editor Marcia Angell. "The great majority of 'new' drugs are not new at all but merely variations of older drugs already on the market."[13]

Due at least in part to the DTC barrage, Americans seem to believe that if they have a symptom, there has to be a drug that can make it disappear. Further, it would not be easy for most physicians to convince patients that their services were worthwhile if they did not prescribe at least *one* drug for new problems addressed at each office visit. Decreasing their utilization of pharmaceutical drugs is not an ideal business strategy for physicians in today's environment. The way HMO medicine is set up supports this situation; it is simply impractical for physicians to take the time needed to thoroughly disclose all the possible side effects of each drug they are prescribing in an office visit that lasts just a few minutes— let alone report side effects to the FDA. In this fast-paced system, there is neither time nor money to provide truly informed health care, let alone genuine healing.

So, where do we stand today? Patients and physicians alike have been taught to reflexively turn to pharmaceutical drugs to manage most health issues. Patients are conditioned to stream into their physicians' offices asking about the latest "purple pill," and physicians are conditioned on all sides to provide it. Everybody knows about the purple pill, and no one wants to be deprived of the wonderful benefits the pill is promised to deliver in TV, radio, magazine, and billboard advertising. At the same time, no one wants to face the fact that this same innocent little purple pill—to give a typical example—also increases the risk for osteoporosis by 45 percent and senile dementia by 18 percent if taken over the long term, or that the pill makes it difficult to digest food properly because there's no longer acid secreted into the stomach, or that it seriously retards the absorption of vitamin B12, calcium, and iron.[14]

Do you still think that little purple pill is such a good idea?

There's a pill for everything! Or so says Big Pharma

Too many of us *do believe* it's a good idea. But just how does pharmaceutical fundamentalism work as a belief system? Try on these affirmations:

Not to worry—our scientific brilliance will take care of your health, even if you don't!

This unspoken assumption, this singular fallacy of our time, has led to the monstrous growth of a medical-industrial complex that feeds off of our poor self-care. Somewhere out there is a pill for every medical condition known to man and almost every imaginable symptom. We are a nation that has learned to depend on silver-bullet solutions for our health problems.

There's really no need to watch what you eat!

Just use Pepcid AC or Zantac to relieve symptoms of heartburn or indigestion. In fact, if you believe DTC ads, you could anticipate these symptoms and take the drugs prophylactically when you know you're going to overindulge.

Don't concern yourself too much about your high cholesterol! In fact, you don't really need to exercise, lose a few pounds, or watch your diet to prevent arteriosclerosis.

You can always take a statin drug such as Lipitor, Crestor, Pravachol, Lescol, Mevacor, Zocor, Vytorin, or many others, even with their record of side effects ranging from muscle injury to liver and kidney dysfunction. You can take them despite the fact that cholesterol is probably *not* the primary cause of heart disease—a thesis substantively supported by Gary Taubes's exhaustively researched study of the politics and deceptions of the faulty lipid hypothesis, *Good Calories, Bad Calories*.[15]

How far can it go? Well, an article published in the *British Medical Journal* in June 2003 suggested that everyone over the age of 55 take what was termed "the Polypill."[16] This pill included a statin drug, three antihypertensive drugs, aspirin, and folic acid. The idea was to prevent the complications of arteriosclerosis by prophylactically treating everyone, whether at risk or not. Maybe it would have been easier to just put it in our water supply as we do with chlorine and fluoride!

With ideas like these floating around in our medical noo-sphere, it should come as little surprise that, as Greg Critser tells us in *Generation Rx*, baby boomers and their offspring have become the most medicated generation in history. In Critser's words, there are pills that "do everything from guarding us against our excesses of drink, food, and tobacco, to increasing our children's performance at school, to jump-starting our own productivity at work, to extending our very time on this mortal soil." Starting out at $10 billion in 1980, total spending on drugs is now about $200 billion per year, and some authorities predict that the amount will double by 2011. By comparison, we spend $10 billion on going to the movies and about $40 billion on books, expenditures that increase just modestly each year.

Pharmaceutical company ties to Congress

"Over the past two decades," wrote Marcia Angell in *The Truth About the Drug Companies*, "the pharmaceutical industry has moved very far from its original high purpose of discovering and producing useful new drugs. Now primarily a marketing machine to sell drugs of dubious benefit, this industry uses its wealth and power to co-opt every institution that might stand in its way, including the U.S. Congress, the FDA, academic medical centers, and the medical profession itself." Like me, you're probably not going to be shocked to discover that Washington politicians routinely go out of their way to support the pharmaceutical industry.

Take the Bayh-Dole Act of 1980 for one example, which made it easier for drug companies to use research discoveries originating from publicly funded laboratories to develop patented drugs.[17] Four years later, the Hatch-Waxman Act greased the slide for cheaper generics to find their way to the market—which at first glance seems to favor you and me—but the act also made it easier for drug companies to get extensions on their patent monopolies.[18] In 1992, Congress passed the Prescription Drug User Fee Act, which resulted in a "clientized" Food and Drug Administration. This one allowed pharmaceutical companies to pay "user fees" in order to expedite the review of their new drugs, thereby loosening and speeding up regulatory processes.[19] Of course, this made it less expensive to test drugs, allowed them to get to market earlier, and enabled profits to come sooner. And let's not forget that pharmaceutical companies fund their own tests for submission to the FDA, which also enables them to design the trial methodology and even provide interpretations of the resulting data that diminish unwanted results and magnify supposed benefits.

Because of all this haste to bring new "miracle" cures into the mainstream (and to line the pockets of Pharma with bigger profits), we have brought far too many drugs into practice prematurely, only to recall them later when they were found to be dangerous or even deadly. Aside from those we have covered here, well-publicized examples of drugs removed from the market include Seldane, thalidomide, phen/fen, Lotronex, Propulcid, Duract, Posicor, Raxar, and Hismanal. These cases are well documented in such books as *The Truth About the Drug Companies*, *Generation Rx*, *Side Effects*,[20] and *Our Daily Meds*.[21]

On some occasions, pharmaceutical companies have brought demonstrably unsafe drugs to market knowingly and deceitfully, making a mockery of FDA and congressional oversight of the industry. For example, *Side Effects*, by former *Boston Globe* reporter Alison Bass, documents how GlaxoSmithKline was convicted of burying evidence showing that its top-selling antidepressant, Paxil, was ineffective for children and possibly harmful to them by engaging in the "deliberate, systematic practice of suppressing unfavorable research results." This is one of many similar cases of evidence suppression in the literature.

The bottom line is that the relationship between Washington and the pharmaceutical industry is incestuous. Pharmaceutical lobbyists have infiltrated deep into the halls of Congress; they now number half a dozen lobbyists on hand for every congressperson and spend over $150 million a year, making Big Pharma the Capitol's largest lobby. What else explains why drugs cost 30 to 60 percent more in the U.S. than in other countries, forcing seniors to ride buses to Mexico and Canada to purchase the same medications? What else explains why Congress passed a law in 2003 that prohibits Medicare, the largest buyer of prescription drugs, from negotiating prices through bulk purchases? What else explains why Dr. Marcia Angell was disinvited from President Obama's inaugural Health Care Summit, but Billy Tauzin, CEO of Pharmaceutical Research and Manufacturers of America (PhRMA), was present? Pharma is simply promoting its own financial interests; the problem is that all too often, Congress and the rest of the government is looking the other way.

Pharmaceutical company ties to physicians

Big Pharma long ago also crossed an ethical line in its determination to virtually bribe physicians to use its products. And it's got the cash to do it. All told, Pharma spends over $20 billion each year on drug promotion; $5 billion is spent on DTC ads, leaving a lot for its main target—the already overwhelmed physicians. One study found that pharmaceutical companies spend between $8,000 and $15,000 annually to reach each practicing physician. But in another, more recent review of this subject published in the January 2008 issue of *PLoS Medicine* (the Public Library of Science online is the only major medical journal that does *not* accept advertising from drug companies), investigators took a more critical look at this estimate and determined that this number is more like $61,000 per physician![22]

Today's doctors are tripping over the drug industry everywhere they turn. Pharma sponsors most continuing medical education classes for physicians. Drug ads pervade medical journals. And drug reps are practically a fixture in the daily lives of doctors. "There is no way to exaggerate how much a part of some doctors' daily lives drug reps have become," wrote Marcia Angell in January 2009 in the *New York Review of Books*. "A typical doctor is visited by several every week, and doctors in high-prescribing specialties may be visited by a dozen in one day."[23] On par with the ratio of Pharma lobbyists to members of Congress, the ratio of drug salespeople to doctors is now about one to six.

As a practicing physician, I can assure you that my colleagues and I are bombarded daily with commercial information about drugs that depicts itself as "scientific" but is obviously biased—in other words, intentionally confusing. Vehicles of this information include our own finest medical journals and reputable websites such as PubMed, not to mention pharmaceutical drug representatives and mailed advertising from drug companies. Much of the time, it is impossible to know whether the information we are getting is evidence based or primarily an advertisement whose purpose is to sell product.

Sometime, leaf through a peer-reviewed medical journal such as the *Journal of the American Medical Association* or the *New England Journal of Medicine*; you'll discover that more pages are dedicated to pharmaceutical ads than to medical content. Can there be any doubt as to whether these and other prestigious medical journals are also influenced by companies paying handsome prices to advertise in their journals? Is it possible that this conflict of interest could have an effect when it comes to accepting or rejecting articles submitted for publication? You bet it is. Perhaps this explains the lame articles I've noted over the years in some of the most respected journals, as well as why certain other articles are rejected for publication for reasons that baffle the intelligent mind.

I was further shocked to learn that some pharmaceutical company research is designed, collected, interpreted, and disseminated by the company's *marketing* division rather than its research department. These studies are called *seeding studies* and are normally deployed after drugs are on the market, with the objective of demonstrating additional uses or advantages over competitors, or simply to get doctors familiar with the product. Results of some of these studies are published in the major peer-reviewed scientific medical journals. Seeding trials are harmful because the motives for doing the trial are concealed, and the scientific question often posed usually has little if any merit except to promote the company's particular product. Aside from the deception that clinically important scientific research is being undertaken, the real victims of these trials are the patients who are put at risk of side effects for no reason other than to increase sales of the drug in question.

The August 19, 2008, issue of the American College of Physicians' *Annals of Internal Medicine* contains an editorial on an article about a Merck seeding study that was previously published in 2003 in that prestigious journal. In this study, which involved 600 investigators and 2,785 patients, Merck's "scientists" compared its drug Vioxx with its strongest competitor, naproxen.[24] This information came to light when a number of e-mails and internal Merck documents became fair game as part of the discovery process of a civil suit involving the cardiovascular safety of Vioxx. It was only then that the primary purpose of this clinical trial—to introduce a new drug in a crowded therapeutic class—was revealed.

Pharmaceutical control over physicians goes beyond influences on their medical training and continuing education, as well as the billions spent on print advertising to doctors. For example, the *New York Times* published an exposé on May 9, 2007, about how two large pharmaceutical companies, Amgen and Johnson & Johnson, were at the time paying hundreds of millions of dollars to doctors every year in return for the doctors' giving their patients a set of three closely related drugs used to treat anemia caused by chemotherapy or kidney failure. The article revealed that one practice of six cancer doctors in the Pacific Northwest had received $2.7 million from Amgen for prescribing $9 million worth of the drugs in the previous year. This may sound exorbitant, but the two companies selling these products grossed a staggering $10 billion that year; in fact, these drugs represented the single biggest pharmaceutical expense for Medicare at that time. Amazingly, the *Times* also reported on FDA research that was unable to find solid scientific evidence to support drug company claims that these medications either improve quality of life or extend survival.[25]

Clearly, Big Pharma's budgets have room for promoting new drugs at the level of a few hundred million dollars a year. But if the drugs were really that helpful, one would think it might not be necessary to entice physicians to prescribe them by giving them what looks like a kickback. The drugs would simply be in great demand by doctors and the public because of their great efficacy.

In light of all this evidence and so much more, many physicians now think twice when a new drug or technology is approved by the FDA and becomes available in clinical practice. They are, of course, keenly interested in deepening the armamentarium of therapeutic modalities that can help the ill, and they're willing to work hard to keep up with the latest scientific research. However, they've learned the hard way that they cannot trust that pharmaceutical companies will disclose all the information they have about the potential side effects of their products. These days, most of my colleagues and I are becoming more interested in what is *not known or not disclosed* about new drugs than what is known. As Marcia Angell reported in her January 2009 *New York Review of Books* article, "Many drugs that are assumed to be effective are probably no better than placebo, but there is no way to know because negative results are hidden."

Pharmaceutical company ties to medical institutions

A medical school faculty's success is measured in part by its ability to raise funds to pay for research projects, salaries, and its teaching programs. Surprise! It turns out that a significant percentage of these funds is provided by the pharmaceutical industry, understandably eager to pay for research needed to bring a new drug to market. And because the industry is footing the bill, it often reserves the right to supervise the interpretation of data and make final decisions on whether results of a scientific study will be published. It also follows that physicians in training at such institutions, who are mentored by those same researchers, are taught to think in terms of specific pharmacological solutions to every medical problem.

A Harvard Medical School study published in the October 2007 issue of *JAMA* surveyed 459 department heads at 125 U.S. medical schools and 15 of the biggest independent teaching hospitals. It discovered that an amazing 67 percent of medical school and teaching hospital departments and 60 percent of department heads personally received money from or enjoyed some type of financial relationship with the pharmaceutical industry.[26] Eric Campbell, the lead author of the study, stated that industry cash commonly flows to individual physicians, scientists, medical schools, medical practices, people on FDA panels, and even institutional review boards that approve medical scientific studies.

Let's look at a few more examples of how corrupting this money can be.

In her 2009 book *Our Daily Meds,* former *New York Times* reporter Melody Petersen uses the case of the drug Neurontin, manufactured by Pfizer, to make what Marcia Angell called "a broad, convincing indictment of the pharmaceutical industry" in her January 2009 *New York Review of Books* article.

Neurontin had originally been approved for a very narrow use: controlling epilepsy seizures. In her book, Petersen traces how Pfizer paid medical academics to put their names on articles extolling Neurontin for unrelated uses, including insomnia, bipolar disease, migraines, and hot flashes. They also funded conferences at which these new uses were promoted. Before long, Pfizer had leveraged these "KOLs" (key opinion leaders) to create a blockbuster drug, reaching sales of $2.7 billion by 2003. This story has a familiar ending: In a case closely watched by Petersen for the *Times*, Pfizer eventually agreed to pay $430 million to the government, pleading guilty to charges of illegal marketing.[27]

Another notorious case is that of Joseph Biederman, chief of pediatric psychopharmacology at Massachusetts General Hospital and professor of psychiatry at Harvard Medical School, who has published hundred of papers on attention deficit hyperactivity disorder (ADHD). In large part due to his research, he claimed that children once thought to have ADHD actually have pediatric bipolar disorder. This controversial theory was proposed at a time when it was unheard of for young children to be diagnosed with this disorder, but his research led to a controversial 40-fold increase in the diagnosis. Then in 2008, congressional investigators revealed that Biederman had received $1.6 million from drug companies—including those who made the drugs he advocated for children with bipolar disorder. Experts quoted in the *New York Times* the same year stated that Biederman's own studies of these drugs were "largely inconclusive."[28]

Big Pharma's bottom line: patent or no patent?

Many natural and inexpensive drug therapies and nutraceuticals never make it into mainstream medical practice, for a simple reason: By law, natural products found in the human body, including hormones (such as estradiol, progesterone, testosterone), enzymes, and nutrients (such as vitamin B_{12}, folic acid, and thiamine), cannot be patented in their natural form. Without a patent, drugmakers won't be able to corner the market with a new product, and therefore they can't justify spending the dollars needed for clinical trials and for getting it in front of physicians. (However, it should be noted that natural substances may be altered enough that they can be patented, as in the case of Provera, a patented progesterone-like synthetic compound that is prescribed by physicians as part of hormone replacement therapy.)

When you bear in mind that it costs pharmaceutical companies in the realm of $500 million to bring a new drug or synthetic nutrient or hormone to market, it is fiscally unrealistic to expect any company to commercialize a nonpatentable product. Anyone who paid for the clinical research necessary to get the FDA to approve a natural product would be, in effect, donating his work to humanity. Of course, nutraceutical companies are permitted to sell their nonpatentable natural products without first carrying out clinic research; that's because these products are not classed as drugs—not yet, anyway—and therefore remain unregulated by the FDA. At the same, these companies cannot legally claim that their products have value as specific medical treatments.

Op-ed contributor and cancer journalist Ralph Moss wrote in the *New York Times* on April 1, 2007, "We could make faster progress against cancer by changing the way drugs are developed. In the current system, if a promising compound can't be patented, it is highly unlikely ever to make it to market—no matter how well it performs in the laboratory. The development of new cancer drugs is crippled as a result." He continued, "In 2004, Johns Hopkins researchers discovered that an off-the-shelf compound called 3-bromopyruvate could arrest the growth of liver cancer in rats. The results were dramatic; moreover, the investigators estimated that the cost to treat patients would be around seventy cents per day. Yet, three years later, no major drug company has shown interest in developing this drug for human use."

Moss went on to say, "[A]nother readily available industrial chemical, dichloroacetate, was found by researchers at the University of Alberta to shrink tumors in laboratory animals by up to 75 percent. However, as a university news release explained, dichloroacetate is not patentable, and the lead researcher is concerned that it may be difficult to find funding from private investors to test the chemical. So the university is soliciting public donations to finance a clinical trial."

Finally, Moss reported, "The hormone melatonin, sold as an inexpensive food supplement in the United States, has repeatedly been shown to slow the growth of various cancers when used in conjunction with conventional treatments. Paolo Lissoni, an Italian oncologist, helped write more than 100 articles about this hormone and conducted numerous clinical trials. But when I visited him at his hospital in Monza in 2003, he was in deep despair over the pharmaceutical industry's total lack of interest in his treatment approach. He has published nothing on the topic since then."[29]

Whose responsibility is it, then, to provide life-saving research when no profits are to be had? Wouldn't it logically fall to our publicly funded institutions to go after such opportunities on behalf of the American public? I believe strongly that the NIH should be funding research on natural substances such as 3-bromopyruvate, dichloroacetate, and melatonin, and making sure that these inexpensive and potentially life-extending natural substances can be taken to clinical trials and brought into clinical practice if they are found to be useful. In a health care system that does not operate entirely according to commercial values, drugs would be judged on their scientific merit alone rather than on their ability to be patented and generate profits.

How could a situation like this develop? What is stopping the NIH from sponsoring scientific research to test these natural substances in clinical trials? Why should the University of Alberta need to look for private funding to finance a clinical trial on dichloroacetate? Hopefully Washington's new interest in comparative effectiveness research will address such questions.

Daniel Haley's book *Politics in Healing* details ten such cases of natural, nontoxic cancer treatments, most of great promise, that were either ignored or directly suppressed by the same establishment that promotes the toxic cancer treatments currently dominant in that field.[30]

Pharma creates a new category: the "worried well"

The practice of relying on medications to prevent disease has led to the adoption of a wide range of pharmaceutical drugs for what has been termed *the worried well*. In June 2005, *Seattle Times* staff writers Susan Kelleher and Duff Wilson wrote a series of articles titled "Suddenly Sick."[31] They concluded that the pharmaceutical industry has, in its greed and arrogance, managed to change the definitions of many diseases such as hypertension, obesity, female sexual dysfunction, and osteoporosis. It accomplished this by extending the boundaries of each definition so that more people are considered to be sick.

For example, they reported that in May 2003, an NIH panel reviewed the definition of hypertension. Prior to this time, the high limit of normal blood pressure, called *systolic* blood pressure, was 140 mm of mercury; the lower number, called *diastolic* blood pressure, was less than 90 mm of mercury. The panel, however, concluded that from then on, blood pressures above 120 systolic and 80 diastolic should be treated. They made up a new term, *prehypertension,* for people with blood pressure between 120 and 140 systolic and between 80 and 90 diastolic.

Investigation of this NIH panel revealed that 9 of its 11 members had ties to pharmaceutical companies as paid consultants, paid speakers, and/or grant recipients. Some of these individuals had ties to as many as 15 different pharmaceutical companies.

As might be predicted, the pharmaceutical industry warmly accepted the recommendations of this "prestigious" panel when it supported the use of drugs to treat prehypertension. The drugmakers promptly began an extensive advertising campaign to promote sales of their expensive patented antihypertensive drugs. This small change in the defining criteria for hypertension resulted in billions of dollars in increased sales of drugs every year. Patients and their insurance companies spent $16.3 billion for antihypertensive medications in 2004. This was up $3 billion from just three years before.

On the other hand, a study titled *Antihypertensive and Lipid-Lowering Treatment to Prevent Heart Attack Trial,* also known as the ALLHAT study, was conducted between 1994 and 2002 by the National Heart, Lung, and Blood Institute section of the NIH and included data from 600 separate medical practices.[32] It was the largest clinical trial published on the subject of drug treatment for hypertension and included more than 42,000 patients. These investigators demonstrated the superiority of time-tested, inexpensive thiazide-type diuretics in preventing cardiovascular disease over all of the newer and far more expensive antihypertensive drugs. The ALLHAT study concluded that diuretics should be the drugs of choice for first-step antihypertensive therapy. Only for the occasional patient who cannot take a diuretic did they recommend considering the far more expensive calcium channel blockers or ACE inhibitors that remain on patent. They also emphasized the importance of lifestyle in managing hypertension.

Sounds good, at first glance—or at least like an improvement over using channel blockers and ACE inhibitors. And if diuretics were innocuous, it might be a good idea to consider treating people with high-normal blood pressure quite freely with them. However, consider that the thiazide diuretics have several potentially serious side effects. First of all, this class of drugs causes the body to lose potassium. Unless potassium is replaced, this can cause serious or even fatal cardiac rhythm disturbances, profound weakness, and gastrointestinal symptoms. Physicians must test their patients' potassium levels regularly. Even then, it is not uncommon for levels to be too high or too low. This can lead to life-threatening problems.

Thiazide diuretics also cause a loss of magnesium in most people. This is well documented in hundreds of articles in the mainstream medical journals, but most physicians don't often measure for magnesium, especially intracellularly, where 99 percent of it is concentrated in the body. Low magnesium levels have been documented to elevate blood pressure, cause serious cardiac-rhythm disorders, cause muscle weakness, aggravate asthma, and even cause seizures. If this isn't enough to scare you, consider that this family of diuretics is well known to increase cholesterol levels, which we all know about, and in addition cause insulin resistance, which can lead to elevated blood sugar and to Type 2 diabetes, with all of its complications. Finally, it can raise serum uric acid levels, which can predispose the patient to attacks of gout. Does it still sound like taking a diuretic for what is arguably "normal" blood pressure—i.e., "prehypertension"—is a good idea? Every single antihypertensive drug on the market has its share of potentially dangerous side effects. Thiazide diuretics may work quite well and save money, but they are still far from ideal. It is also important to point out, of course, that *none of the pharmaceutical drugs on the market treat the underlying cause of elevated blood pressure.*

Kelleher and Wilson went on to report a story about how the criteria used to diagnose osteoporosis have changed. This is another example of the new phenomenon of the worried well, also known by some as the Suddenly Sick Syndrome. Once again, we see a convenient vagueness in what experts say about when treatment is indicated. At what point would it be wise to begin taking extra steps to prevent fractures of the spine or hip? And what treatment is most appropriate? Of course, the answer depends on what you are trying to accomplish.

Kelleher and Wilson proposed that a new disease has been invented—preosteoporosis, or *osteopenia*. People with osteopenia have bone density readings that are not outside the accepted range of normal but are in the lower portion of the normal range. These people—as part of the worried well—have only a slightly increased risk for fractures. However, the thinking is that if their bone densities happen to be on the downtrend, they could possibly be at a significantly high risk for developing true osteoporosis. This is a big "if." Consequently, many people who have a relatively normal risk for fracture have been told they have a disease, when what they actually have is merely a measurement that might become abnormal at some future time, should their bone density drop below the lower limit of normal.

Many authorities are now proposing that women with osteopenia be treated "preventively" with drugs to "make sure" that no further deterioration is likely to occur and result in a fracture. Of course, this is precisely the stance that the pharmaceutical industry itself has taken. And you'll not be surprised to learn that it has led to billions of dollars in sales every year of the drugs used in the treatment of osteoporosis. This kind of thinking may sound logical, but it is clearly not the evidence-based science that mainstream medicine purports to practice. Whom do you suppose was responsible for bringing this policy into clinical practice?

The National Osteoporosis Foundation estimates that there are 10 million people with osteoporosis and another 44 million with osteopenia. This represents 55 percent of people over the age of 50. It is noteworthy that this organization receives backing from the pharmaceutical industry. Hmmm . . .

If the drugs used to treat osteopenia were entirely safe and not expensive, this might not be such an important issue. But all of the bisphosphonates (Fosamax, Actonel, Didronel, Boniva, Aredia, Zometa, Reclast, and Skelid) can have dreadful consequences that include gastrointestinal irritation, ulcers of the esophagus, skin rash, low blood calcium, atrial fibrillation, painful muscles and joints. It can also lead to *osteonecrosis* of the jaw, a terrible condition that involves serious deterioration of the jawbone and leads to the loss of many teeth as well as considerable pain. In the May/June 2008 issue of the *Journal of Orthopaedic Trauma*, physicians from Cornell University wrote, "Increasing evidence suggests long-term alendronate [Fosamax] use may overly suppress bone metabolism, limiting repair of microdamage and creating risk for insufficiency fractures."[33] Recent studies revealed that when bisphosphonates are used to prevent bone loss in patients with cancer, the incidence of osteonecrosis of the jaw is a staggering 3 to 12 percent.[34, 35] These "side effects" are not only disabling and unpleasant, but are sometimes fatal.

The pharmaceutical companies that manufacture these drugs don't highlight how bisphosphonates work. The truth is, if the information from the drug companies making these drugs is correct, they are actually a form of chemotherapy. There are two specialized cells in bone that work in homeostatic balance to regulate bone density. Osteoblasts lay down new bone, and osteoclasts remove old bone. Bisphosphonates kill osteoclasts. This is a novel way to increase bone density, but only long-term studies will determine if increasing bone density with old bone is a good idea.

Of course, there's a safer but nonpatentable way to go: Generally speaking, people with osteopenia and osteoporosis can be treated very effectively by trying a few simple and inexpensive strategies before considering potentially dangerous drug therapy. Lifestyle approaches such as doing weight-bearing exercise, supplementing with small amounts of calcium and micronutrients, consuming foods high in calcium and essential fatty acids (such as flaxseed or fish oil), taking in sufficient amounts of vitamins D_3 and K_2 and strontium, reducing stress, and getting adequate sleep are the most effective and safest ways to restore and maintain healthy bones.

It is also important to assess levels of thyroid, adrenal, and sex hormones, as imbalances of these hormones can lead to osteoporosis. It is only common sense that we avoid drugs that can cause osteoporosis, such as cortisone derivatives, SSRI antidepressants, drugs that block acid production in the stomach (such as Prilosec, Aciphex, Nexium, Protonix, and Prevacid), Dilantin, Heparin, Coumadin, Lasix, methotrexate, caffeine, and tobacco.[36]

Another important factor beyond basic medical school training and exposure to advertising encourages many of our physicians to buy into the Suddenly Sick Syndrome. Think about it: Our doctors are clinicians, not scientists. They are on the front lines doing their best to use the latest and best treatments for us. They depend on a wide range of educational resources to guide them to the most effective treatment plans in clinical practice. These resources include their long and rigorous education, studies from research scientists and pharmaceutical and technology companies, and their own common sense. They also depend on government to act as a watchdog over profit-hungry purveyors of drugs and technologies. It is expecting a lot from physicians who are overworked and doing their best to keep up with the complicated technical advances in scientific and pharmaceutical research to find the time to develop the expertise to set standards of care for hundreds of diseases.

In the end, the way in which physicians practice medicine is directly related to what they are taught. Don't believe for a minute that what they are taught is necessarily factual. As we have seen here, a significant amount of the information they learn comes from medical research that is directly influenced by what generates sales for Pharma. As has also been presented earlier, much of what is published is not truly evidence based—and, in the final analysis, sometimes turns out to be just another form of creative advertising.

To conclude this chapter, consider the hormone replacement therapy (HRT) story. Until recently, HRT treatments with the drug Prempro had for several decades been standard care for women going through menopause. Prempro was also touted by its manufacturer, Wyeth, not only as the established treatment for menopause, but also as an antiaging strategy that would help reduce wrinkles as well as reduce heart attacks, strokes, and probably breast cancer.

Yet as far back as 1987, an article by C. Bengstsson in the March issue of *Maturitas* documented that the incidence of breast cancer was 59 percent higher in women on HRT. At first, no one believed this study could be correct. Then, in July 2002, researchers at the NIH concluded that HRT using Prempro posed a significant risk of heart attack, stroke, and cancer. Their lengthy study of 16,000 women was planned to last until 2005 but was abruptly stopped because of the negative data about side effects. At the time, six million women were using Prempro! Now it is common knowledge that the effects of HRT on the heart are negative—that is, it *increases* the incidence of heart attacks. There is also evidence showing that, for the first time ever, there was a sudden drop of 7 percent in the rate of breast cancer that coincided with a drop in HRT usage in the year 2002–3.

Cases like these—and there are many more—are evidence that the medical profession, the FDA, and pharmaceutical companies have some serious soul-searching to do. So too does the majority of the American public that has been so gullibly accepting medical standards of practice influenced by Big Pharma.

Considering its record of influence-buying, deceptive advertising, and compromised research, as well as its many public scandals—not to mention its unprecedented levels of profit each year—there can be no doubt that Big Pharma has big karma.

Six

Wellness, Prevention, and Healing: The New Direction for Medicine

Health is a state of complete physical, mental, and social well-being and not merely the absence of disease or infirmity.

—World Health Organization

The biggest problem with the U.S. health-care system is that it has long been designed to respond to illness rather than prevent it.

—*Time*, "America's Health Checkup," December 1, 2008

When we're sick, most of us will do whatever it takes to get rid of our symptoms; our disease care system is, after all, built around capitalizing upon this simple impulse. The implicit trajectory of today's medical technology and pharmaceuticals is to one day fulfill this desire, overcoming *all* of our symptoms and *every* disease.

Such fanciful science-fiction logic would probably be valid if human health were an advanced engineering problem, the solution to which paid out the highest net profit.

Yet it's not surprising that most Americans accept this approach, for some things in life really are that simple and mechanical:

Experiencing a difficulty? Buy a service or product that solves it and reward the provider with riches. We're the land of the technological quick fix. We *should* expect our scientists and physicians to come up with tricks to relieve our suffering, right? After all, no one *wants* to feel sick.

Unfortunately, human biology is not that simple. Feeling better in the moment is only one part of what an ideal health care system should provide.

Let's take a look at what an advanced health care system should accomplish when it has put a priority on a return to healing.

Getting acquainted with the wellness buffer

The point of fighting disease is easy to appreciate. But the ideal, of course, is that diseases never occur in the first place—and that we remain in optimal health by regularly pursuing healthy lifestyle practices.

We all know about the simple, effective, and inexpensive practices that promote good health through prevention, and we all agree they work. Yet we often find ourselves ignoring them. After all, as *Time* magazine reported in the article cited above, "If you're like 67 percent of Americans, you're currently overweight or obese. If you're like 96 percent of the population, you may not be able to recall the last time you had a salad, since you're one of the hundreds of millions of Americans who rarely eat enough vegetables. And what you do eat, you don't burn off—assuming you're like the 40 percent of us who get no exercise." What's worse, if we look closely, we discover that our current health care system reinforces this ignorance and laziness—in fact, profits from it. We'll also discover that the infrastructure needed to support wellness and prevention simply isn't present in the United States; the commercial interests that drive today's medical care have little to gain from building such an infrastructure.

On the other hand, there's nothing to stop smart business-people from capitalizing just as much on what might be called the *wellness impulse*: the inner urge many of us have to achieve peak health. In his 2002 book *The Wellness Revolution*, economist Paul Zane Pilzer outlined an emerging $200 billion industry he called "the wellness business."[1] The latest edition of the book, *The New Wellness Revolution* (2007), claims that the natural medicine and wellness industry has grown to $500 billion annually, providing ever-increasing entrepreneurial opportunities in natural health, integrative medicine, prevention, nutrition, and much more.

It appears that the worldview conflict at the heart of America's health care dilemma has led to a clash of industries. But what if there were a way to bridge the gap between the two in a single concept?

Consider this: Picture your state of health as a spectrum that extends from one pole on the left—where there is (theoretically) perfect functioning of body, mind, and spirit—to the opposite pole on the right, where death exists. In between these two extremes lies a place where symptoms of dysfunction have not quite yet surfaced but where we have lost some of our perfect functionality. I call this critical zone our *wellness buffer*.

In conventional medicine, this place is usually not on the map. Disease care doesn't get involved in the issue of wellness unless symptoms have developed. Restoring a well-functioning body, mind, or spirit is irrelevant *until* a person has lost the cushion of his wellness buffer, and when a good bit of remediation is now required. A simplified version of the full spectrum between perfect health and death is shown in the diagram below:

The Functional Spectrum of Wellness and Disease

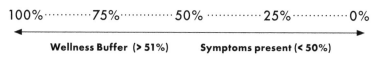

Figure 6.1 The wellness buffer extends from 51 to 100% (perfect health). Symptoms begin to surface only at 50% of functionality, or less.

In today's medicine, the gold standard for diagnosing good health is the act of documenting the absence of signs and symptoms of disease—that is, it's in the business of exploring only 50 percent of the total spectrum! Optimal health is not under investigation; a "clean bill of health" simply means that nothing is severe enough to show evidence of symptoms during a physical examination or in abnormal findings in routine laboratory testing. Such measures don't identify the magnitude or extent of a patient's wellness buffer or how close she may be to theoretical perfect function; nor do they show the patient explicitly how to move toward optimal function once symptoms have disappeared.

It's a matter of paradigm: Today's diagnostics are geared to detect diseases from the middle to the far right end of the spectrum, where the horse is already out of the barn—maladies such as cancer, diabetes, and heart disease. These tests accurately measure the biochemical and physiological function of many organ systems; many sensitively assay the total function of such organs as the heart, lungs, and kidneys. However, as long as the results of these analyses are within the so-called normal range with no overt symptoms present, nothing more will be done.

For example, the ability of the heart to pump blood can be measured by a number called the *ejection fraction*, which defines "normal" values as those between 50 and 62 percent. Most people can function quite well at 50 percent, but it is not as ideal as 62 percent—which indicates more advanced wellness. Physicians are not inclined to treat a patient with an ejection fraction at the low end of normal, in part because drugs and surgery—the only remedies at hand—have the potential to cause severe side effects. Lifestyle strategies in these cases can be very helpful in promoting prevention and increased wellness, but physicians are not trained to deliver this aspect of health care.

The same is true when measuring lung function. Some of these tests are highly sophisticated, and they do in fact measure all the way up to ideal total lung physiology. Again, however, unless there is sufficient loss of function such that lifestyle is impaired, no concentrated effort is made to restore lung function to optimal levels.

To restate: Science has learned that our body's organs have remarkable reserves that protect us from the symptoms of disease, and we can measure the extent of these reserves all the way up to theoretical perfect function. Our functional reserves let us remain symptom free across a good part of the spectrum. All may appear well in our general health right up to the point where we've lost as much as 50 percent of an organ's total reserve function. Until we reach this point of loss, we may have no idea that we're dangerously near the edge of a cliff. To put it numerically: If we are scoring 100, we're perfect in function and in peak health. At 90 or 80 we're not too bad. But if we fall between, say, 70 and 55, we're in danger of losing our remaining buffer and falling off the edge into disease.

We have all heard stories that illustrate this issue. These are the tragic tales about people who had recently gone to their doctor for a routine checkup, including an EKG and routine lab work, and were told they were in good health. Seemingly out of nowhere, within hours to days, they suffered a heart attack and were hospitalized or even died. Do you really think these people were in good health one day, yet seriously ill or even dead the next?

Let us not be fooled by the large but hidden middle ground that spans the distance from perfect functioning to the onset of symptoms. Instead, we should all be working to maintain the optimum amount of reserve protection in our organs. Our most potent defense is a good offense, one based on living a healthy lifestyle.

The Pete Wilson and Tim Russert stories

Pete Wilson was a popular and treasured ABC news anchor and radio broadcaster in the San Francisco Bay Area for more than 30 years. In July 2007, Wilson was scheduled for elective hip replacement surgery at a well-known medical facility in the San Francisco Bay Area. He passed his physical examination, EKG, and routine laboratory work with flying colors. To make a sad story short, Wilson died of a heart attack on the operating table. How could this have happened?

First of all, this story is not that unusual. And yes, he did have state-of-the-art medical screening at a university hospital with an outstanding reputation. You might wonder why his physicians didn't consider that they were dealing with someone over the age of 60 who was a bit overweight, was under considerable stress and anxiety, and was possibly at high risk for heart disease—and therefore delay a major surgical procedure until more in-depth screening tests could be completed.

Wilson must have had an intuition that all was not right with his level of wellness. During the last hour of his final radio broadcast, the day before his surgery, he talked about his worries concerning the surgery with fellow radio talk show host Gene Burns and invited callers to recount their own surgical experiences. It was reported later, after his death, that Wilson had had severe anxiety about his upcoming surgery and had gone the night before to the emergency room because of it.

Yet everything was pronounced "normal," and the deadly surgery was performed the following day.

Wilson had received from a prestigious medical center the standard of care expected by the Medical Board of California. But did he really get the care he needed and deserved? At least two inexpensive and safe, Medicare-approved tests could have been done to screen for occult (i.e., hidden) heart disease. In his case, chances are that both a heart-rate variability test and a test for vascular stiffness would have come out abnormal, as these tests are measures of organ functionality that expose disease when it falls well within the range of the wellness buffer (at the left side of the spectrum). This might well have led to uncovering his underlying critical heart problems and to the proper preventive treatment that had the potential to save him from his destined fatal heart attack. Even so, these are still not standard tests in cases like that of Pete Wilson.

In addition, sending anyone to surgery—especially an elective surgery—when he is in a state of extreme anxiety seems imprudent. This, of course, points to yet another blind spot in the current mechanistic paradigm—the inextricable role of the mind and emotions in health. If this commonsense factor—well understood these days in the emerging scientific field of mind-body medicine—had only been recognized, then Wilson would ideally have been referred for preoperative interactive guided imagery. An extensive literature indicates the benefits of positive imagery before surgery, documenting that when it is employed, there is less blood loss during surgery, less pain afterward, faster healing, and certainly less anxiety throughout the entire process. Nancy Huddleston's book and audiotape titled, *Prepare for Surgery, Heal Faster*, featured nationwide on PBS-TV and now recommended by several leading hospitals, explains how to use relaxation to calm preoperative jitters and to create the biochemistry that enhances healing. It also guides the patient in using visualization and healing imagery, mobilizes the healing power of a support group of family and friends, and even creates a healing role for the anesthesiologist. Ongoing research has shown the efficacy of this system, yet it remains too little known among surgeons trained in the old reductionistic paradigm.

While "routine" testing may work for the majority of patients as screens before surgery, the case of Pete Wilson shows that it obviously does not suffice for all. The art of medicine requires that physicians take time to know each patient as a whole person and use their experience and judgment to determine when the standard one-size-fits-all workup is insufficient.

A second instance is the tragic story of Tim Russert, another beloved broadcast journalist. In his 16th year as moderator of NBC's *Meet the Press*, he died, at 58, of an unexpected heart attack while at work. His physician stated that Russert had ruptured plaque in a major coronary artery that led to its abrupt closure and his sudden demise. Yet Russert had passed a stress EKG test just a couple of months earlier.

Russert was overweight, was under considerable stress, and had an enlarged heart. It had been determined that he had *asymptomatic* arteriosclerotic heart disease (meaning that he was still in the wellness buffer zone). He was being treated with drugs and exercise, a conventional approach that in retrospect was clearly insufficient. Suppressing symptoms without dealing with the underlying causes is unfortunately the standard of "good" medical practice in this setting.

I wonder how many additional risk factors Russert had for premature coronary artery disease and what his doctors might have learned, had he been given a heart-rate variability test and a vascular stiffness test. And what if he had been more aggressively treated for his weight and high stress levels with intensive nutritional counseling and more effective stress-reduction strategies?

The upshot is that if we are to prevent these scenarios, it is important to measure the reserve function of our organ systems—a superior approach compared with simply screening for symptoms of advanced disease without taking preventive action to reverse silently progressing and potentially lethal health problems.

This new style of medicine, called *functional medicine*, exists today and is available as part of the repertoire of the integrative approach. Want to guess why it is not routinely practiced? The above examples indicate that the disease care model has little interest in addressing and dealing with wellness and prevention.

It should now be clearer why good health means much more than simply not having symptoms of disease; nevertheless, we still find ourselves waiting to get sick before seeking medical attention. Today's HMO medicine aggravates this problem by putting pressure on physicians to treat only the physical symptoms of disease, not the underlying health and lifestyle problems that lead us to getting sick—and it gives only lip service to our deeper human needs. In this setting, physicians are rewarded for evaluating and treating us as quickly as possible and with as little support from their specialist colleagues as they can.

And prevention, of course, is not on the agenda.

While functional medicine is an effective way to diagnose and prevent the very early onset of disease, it is generally non-reimbursable by insurance entities such as Medicare and HMOs. Amazingly, Medicare does not even have diagnostic billing codes for most preventive medical services. It states that these kinds of tests or practices are "not indicated." Yet there are often simple and inexpensive ways, as in the cases of Pete Wilson and Tim Russert, to avoid the progression of diseases that can result in very expensive hospitalizations, not to mention death.

One of the most crucial changes needed in today's medical care is reimbursement for preventive, integrative, and wellness strategies from the health care insurance providers. At today's rate of change, it may take a virtual revolution to get it.

Differentiating curing and healing

Let's now revisit a closely related issue that we have only lightly touched upon: the distinction between curing and healing. By our definition, curing is focused on eliminating symptoms. Yet curing symptoms is just the beginning of healing. Genuine healing moves us along toward peak health—not just in organ function but in all functions of body, mind, emotion, and spirit. Healing addresses *all* aspects of our being—just as if these too are "organs" that deserve peak function and, in a real sense, have their own wellness spectrums.

Consider: If there is a purpose or a reason for everything that happens in the universe—as I believe there is—then what would be the value in restoring physical health without learning from the experience of being sick? From this point of view, curing the symptoms of disease alone could be looked upon as having a negative impact on a patient's opportunity for emotional, intellectual, and spiritual growth. If the stimulus to learn is removed with an external fix and we are no longer suffering, how many of us would still seek to learn why we got sick in the first place? That's why the deepest responsibility of an ideal health care system includes guiding us as human beings to ultimate healing as one feature of a spiritual path—a path of personal growth in wisdom and self-knowledge.

Throughout history, ancient healing traditions have always encompassed the responsibility of guiding patients through their life challenges, especially illness; poor health in this context offers insights into the whole person that might otherwise be difficult or even impossible to learn. Illness itself, then, can be regarded as a teacher of wisdom. And wisdom, in turn, teaches us that we must act to prevent illness in the first place through living a life of virtue and loving-kindness that includes healthy lifestyle practices.

The virtuous life in this sense allows us to maintain an optimal position, or *homeostasis*, in the domain of the wellness buffer, with the goal of evolving toward perfection in body-mind-spirit health. No wonder we are witnessing a massive revival of the ancient traditions of healing and the CAM practices that are often derived from them: They teach us that the needs of the whole person are central to the mission of true healing.

Focusing on the whole person is nearly impossible in the current model

Now, let's contrast genuine healing with today's medicine. In our single-minded quest to identify and overcome the symptoms of illness alone, the practice of medicine has become almost unimaginably technical, complicated, impersonal, and fragmented. The myriad of subspecialties, such as cardiology, neurology, gastroenterology, nephrology, and endocrinology, make it nearly impossible for any single person—even a physician specializing in a particular area—to be fully versed in her own field, let alone all fields. No wonder general-practice physicians are often overwhelmed. The managed care system gives them very limited time and resources to figure out which treatments are best, let alone teach patients how to understand what is happening to them and why it is necessary that they receive a given treatment. It becomes tempting to defer to the expertise of the subspecialist most concerned with a particular malady, especially considering his lifetime of devotion to learning the intricacies of his field.

But remember our earlier conclusion: It is not just the amount of knowledge or technique that an expert commands that makes the difference; rather, it's the way knowledge and wisdom are *applied* that determines the best outcome. And this is a function of the humility of the practitioner, as well as her spiritual attainment as an individual and her ability to be authentically present with the patient—that is, to address the *needs of the whole person for healing*, not simply curing the symptoms. That's a crucial lesson I've derived from my experience of four decades of clinical practice.

And here we've come full circle. The services of any given specialist usually cannot be applied for genuine healing without consideration of what is needed by the whole person in the most inclusive context. Each specialist's service must be woven into the fabric of a comprehensive treatment program that often involves several *other* specialists, some of whose services are so technical that a personal relationship with the patient is not even considered because it is not possible or practical. Further, all of the specialties one is struggling to coordinate *still* exclude many of the issues we have identified as crucial to the whole health of a given individual—physical, biochemical, bioenergetic, emotional, environmental, cultural, and spiritual.

The emerging *integral* medicine does, of course, encompass these things. When practicing this new medicine with a goal of providing true healing in such situations, quarterbacking and team-building is crucial. At least in theory, the core responsibility of the primary care physician becomes one of educating and guiding his patients through a complex decision-making process that can involve a multitude of disciplines and specialists.

What about the patient? We are all different, and making the "right" decision often has a lot to do with who we are, what we prefer, and what we can afford, as well as our unique medical and personal situation. To get at that decision, we want to *partner* with our health care practitioners, all of them. And we want our health care practitioners to partner with each other too.

Many primary care doctors would love to pursue collaborations and explorations of this kind. But we have learned in previous chapters that the current system is simply not designed for this. Physicians are generally far too busy to carefully review the medical situation at hand and negotiate a treatment plan with each patient—even within the disease care paradigm. Partnering is critical, but it is rarely possible in clinical settings regulated by a managed health care system that typically offers only ten minutes for each patient visit, and focuses on drugs and surgery to manage symptoms of disease.

Many patients and their families are highly motivated and capable of participating in their own medical research and sharing in the decision-making process that leads to the best and most appropriate treatment options and choices. The Internet has made available a tremendous amount of medical information to physicians and for patients and their families. And this new age of readily accessible highly technical information is leading to an even greater desire by patients for a new, collaborative, and person-centered approach to medicine.

But as the saying goes, we don't always get what we want.

Public surveys reveal
what Americans want from medicine

While most Americans have great respect and even awe for the amazing technology of modern medicine, they are considerably dissatisfied with its lack of success in treating chronic diseases, the safety issues of its drugs and surgeries, its inequities of access, its rising cost, and its depersonalized nature. Americans appreciate that we are living longer than ever before, that some epidemics of childhood diseases have largely been eradicated, and that we are close to bringing the potential wonders of stem cell transplants and gene therapy into clinical practice. Medical technology has accomplished what were once regarded as impossible feats. It would be foolish to discard these brilliant advances. And while Americans are moving toward something—still incompletely defined—that transcends the dire problems of the old disease care model, they still want to include its best features in the new medicine that is evolving.

More than a decade ago, Harvard Medical School's David Eisenberg, MD, documented that health care in America was indeed entering a new era of *integrative medicine,* the predecessor of integral-health medicine. In his two landmark articles—one published in 1993 in *NEJM,* which shocked the medical world, and its 1998 sequel in *JAMA*—he verified a powerful, sustained progression of change.[2, 3]

According to his widely discussed 1998 report, "Alternative medicine use and expenditures increased substantially between 1990 and 1997, attributable primarily to an increase in the proportion of the population seeking alternative therapies, rather than increased visits per patient." He went on to report, "Extrapolations to the US population suggest a 47.3 percent increase in total visits to alternative medicine practitioners, from 427 million in 1990 to 629 million in 1997, *thereby exceeding total visits to all US primary care physicians* [emphasis added]." Further, "Total out-of-pocket expenditures relating to alternative therapies were conservatively estimated at $27 billion, which is comparable with the projected 1997 out-of-pocket expenditures for all U.S. MD services." Here are additional facts that emerged from this stunning research:

- Total visits to CAM providers (629 million) exceeded total visits to all primary care physicians (386 million) in 1997.

- Out-of-pocket expenditures for herbal products and high-dose vitamins in 1997 were estimated at $8 billion.

- An estimated 15 million adults in 1997 took prescription medications concurrently with herbal remedies and high-dose vitamins.

- The majority of CAM therapy users perceived the combination of CAM and conventional care to be superior to either alone (79 percent).

- The majority of CAM therapy users typically saw a medical doctor before or concurrent with their visits to a CAM provider (70 percent) and did not disclose their use of CAM therapy to their medical doctor (63 to 72 percent).

More recent studies, though not as broad in scope, have confirmed the trend. The National Center for Complementary and Alternative Medicine at the NIH released a survey in May 2004 showing that 36 percent of U.S. adults use some form of alternative remedy. Their definition of CAM practices included acupuncture, meditation, the use of herbal supplements, and prayer. When prayer used specifically for health reasons is included in the definition of complementary and alternative medicine, the number of U.S. adults using complementary and alternative medicine rises to 62 percent, the report stated.[4]

A February 2006 *New York Times* article said that the billions that U.S. residents spend annually on alternative and complementary medicine provide the "most telling evidence of Americans' dissatisfaction with traditional health care." According to the

Times, an estimated 48 percent of U.S. adults used at least one alternative or complementary treatment in 2004, compared with 42 percent in 1994. And health care experts maintain that the rate continues to increase "for reasons that have as much to do with increasing distrust of mainstream medicine and the psychological appeal of nontraditional approaches as with the therapeutic properties of herbs or other supplements." Americans who use CAM treatments often have a "sense of disappointment" or "betrayal" related to a "misdiagnosis, an intolerable drug, failed surgery, even a dismissive doctor." Notably, "haggles with insurance providers, conflicting findings from medical studies and news reports of drug makers' covering up product side effects all feed their disaffection," according to the *Times.*[5]

There can be no doubt that conventional medicine is steadily losing market share in the health care business, and Americans are demanding this new medicine with their pocketbooks. We are now spending out of pocket far in excess of $30 billion a year for CAM services, according to the National Center for Complementary and Alternative Medicine.

Although this emerging paradigm shift in America's health care is impressive, its institutional formation is only in its infancy. Fortunately, there is still time to analyze what has happened, adapt to these changes in consumer preference, and step forward with a solution that can creatively merge the best of both conventional and CAM worlds, providing a greater choice of options to prevent disease as well as restore and maintain good health, all across the entire spectrum of health and disease. The story of my own attempt at such a merger begins in the next chapter.

Patients and their families demand integrative care

Most of the public now knows that mainstream medicine can't provide all the right answers. If it did, we would not be so sick, our health care institutions would not be so dysfunctional and costly, and our system of delivery would not be rated behind those of Colombia, Morocco, Chile, and Costa Rica. On the one hand is immense pressure for radical reform of health care delivery; and on the other, a massive interest in new models of health and healing itself, especially through choices that could involve CAM alone or in conjunction with mainstream strategies.

This new era will feature a new breed of health care practitioners who are open to learning, willing to challenge traditionally accepted principles, and committed to exploring eclectic, integrative, or integral approaches for treatment. Many physicians are beginning to embrace this style of practice, and my colleagues and I have been experimenting with these ideas since 1994 through a nonprofit educational foundation, the Health Medicine Forum, in Northern California. I have also brought this style of health care into clinical practice at the Health Medicine Center in Walnut Creek, California.[6]

Nevertheless, despite patients' massive interest in CAM services, integrative services are institutionalized in clinical practices only in isolated cases. At the moment, the most expedient way to obtain an integrative strategy is to work *independently* of the mainstream physician, if one is in charge or involved!

Indeed, it is common for patients to work with CAM practitioners without ever informing their primary care physician. They want the services of both and, understandably, do not want to create an adversarial stance with either. Even if the conventional primary care physician were aware of the patient's use of CAM, resulting in a great deal of CAM input and information from the patient and CAM practitioner, it is simply not practical for physicians working in managed care to deal with all the additional issues or perspectives being raised. Bear in mind that conventional medical training today *still* barely touches upon CAM approaches.

A good example of this dilemma is the treatment of most cancers. Abundant data published in mainstream medical journals documents the fact that the majority of people with advanced cancer search for CAM approaches in addition to their mainstream cancer treatment. This alone strongly suggests that the public has lost considerable confidence in many conventional cancer therapies that essentially limit their focus to the use of surgery, radiation, and chemotherapy. Anyone in this situation, especially if their conventional treatment were not working, would want to know if alternative therapies outside of mainstream medicine might help him. But it is almost impossible to find mainstream physicians who have deep knowledge of both conventional and CAM treatments for cancer. Obviously there is a critical need to coordinate care for these patients through collaboration. Indeed, a great deal is at stake for the patient!

Take, for example, the known effectiveness of surgery and chemotherapy for breast cancer. And let's assume for the sake of argument that these conventional treatments extend life on the average by about 25 percent—though one could make a good case that they are less effective than that. Now compare this with a startling finding published in the *Journal of Clinical Oncology* in June 2007. In a study of about 1,500 women who had been treated conventionally for breast cancer an average of two years earlier, the researchers found that women who stuck to a healthy diet consisting of lots of fruits and vegetables and were moderately active with physical exercise had a *44 percent* lower risk of dying within a ten-year period.[7, 8]

On the prevention side, one study published June 8, 2007, in the *American Journal of Clinical Nutrition* reported that use of vitamin D supplements is associated with a 60 to 77 percent lower risk of cancer.

Combine this with the results of a study that David Spiegel from Stanford Medical Center published in the *Lancet* in 1989.[9] He compared the longevity of stage-four breast cancer patients who were treated with imagery, support groups, and emotional support, as well as conventional medical treatment, with that of patients who received only the conventional medical treatment. Women in the latter, control group, who had no further cancer treatment options, lived the expected 19 months. Those in the former treatment group lived an average of 37 months. This is a nearly 100 percent increase in survival!

Despite the fact that we need further research to more precisely clarify the role that imagery, group therapy, and psychotherapy play in treating patients with cancer, Spiegel remained convinced that it is "very clear" that support groups provide benefits to cancer patients and should be an important part of their treatment. Doesn't this information make you wonder why the medical profession has not focused on the use of lifestyle strategies primarily, and the use of all other medical treatments secondarily, when managing patients with cancer?

It would therefore also seem like a no-brainer that having a team of health care practitioners from a wide range of disciplines work together with patients would be the most ideal way to support them. However, it is most unusual for mainstream and CAM practitioners to work side by side as partners and collaborate with one another. Can you imagine how satisfying it would be for patients to openly meet with their surgeon, oncologist, CAM practitioners, social worker, psychologist, bodyworkers, and others—sometimes even in the same room at the same time? And to have a single person act as the quarterback, or guide, to coordinate the work of all these disciplines? In the next chapter I present an innovation that permits this very process, which I call *Healing Circles*.

The urgent need for birthing a new paradigm of medicine

The American public is without a doubt demanding a "new medicine." The health care they seek is integrative, holistic, person-centered, and focused on prevention and wellness—a medical model in which nutrition, natural therapies, a healthy lifestyle, a clean environment, a less stressful work environment, and a meaningful purpose in life are cornerstones.

We also want and need a personal relationship with our physicians. It is not acceptable that physicians focus on treating symptoms with technology alone or that they do not work in collaboration with other modalities of healing. The emerging new style of health care also requires that physicians spend enough time with us to develop a sacred space within which we can be deeply heard and develop an honest, personal connection. Further, we want our health care practitioners and health care system to put much more emphasis on prevention, including the building of an infrastructure to support a culture of prevention, wellness, and the pursuit of peak health.

Today we want genuine physician-healers. We want them to be authentic. We prefer that they be vulnerable and be willing to accept that not knowing how to solve difficult health issues is okay with us. And we want to be included in their decision-making processes that will affect the way we experience and manage our illness.

We also realize that it takes time to find the deeper meaning in illness. We are interested in addressing more than the simple physical misfortune and psychological challenge imposed by illness. We want to know more about why we became ill in the first place, how it affects our whole life, and any spiritual lessons that may be related to our particular disease.

We are beginning to understand the difference between curing and healing, and we want to address both. We care about curing our symptoms because we do not want to suffer. Yet simply curing the body's symptoms does not in itself heal the soul. Healing involves a consideration of who we are, how our illness relates to our life story, and how our life interrelates with our society and culture, and with everything in the universe.

Seven

The Birth of the Health Medicine Movement

Medicine is in trouble. Each of us carries the responsibility to help craft a new, more fitting map. . . . Simply by taking time to consider an integral perspective, we are helping to hospice an old paradigm that is ceasing to work. In so doing, we must be gentle with ourselves, with each other, and with a system of medicine that is struggling with its very existence.

—Marilyn Schlitz, President, Institute of Noetic Sciences, from the introduction to *Consciousness and Healing*

Integral medicine is in its infancy. As such, the medical and health-care practitioners who are helping to forge an integral practice are on a voyage of incredible discovery, arguably one of the most important that the millennia-old profession of medicine has ever made.

—Ken Wilber, from the foreword to *Consciousness and Healing*

I'll never forget my first impression of Chinese acupuncture as a young student at Duke University Medical School. One night, a group of us found ourselves riveted to a television as we watched a Chinese man having open chest surgery while casually eating an orange. We were breathless with disbelief! This image planted in me one of the seeds that would lead me not only to embrace a new model of medicine, but to also bring it into clinical practice—as we'll see in the next two chapters.

Since those naïve days in the 1960s, the field of complementary and alternative medicine (CAM) has grown at a tremendous pace, along with the allied effort to create an expanded model of health care delivery. By the 1980s, practitioners of the new *holistic* and natural approaches to healing had become a fixture of American life. Their presence and popularity engendered the growth of research into such new fields as clinical nutrition and herbs, homeopathy and naturopathy, Oriental and Ayurvedic medicine, chiropractic medicine and bodywork, and the new field of mind-body medicine, which focuses on the role of intention and consciousness in health. Coming up from the cutting edge of biomedical research were philosophically compatible advances such as orthomolecular medicine, psychoneuroimmunology, bioenergetics, functional medicine, and epigenetics. New research also began to reveal much more about the role of environmental toxins in human health. Corresponding to these discoveries, a movement toward self-care and personal responsibility for health arose among more intelligent Americans, emphasizing a philosophy of healing, wellness, and prevention over allopathic disease care, and focusing on lifestyle factors such as natural foods, frequent exercise, psychological integration, and spiritual practice. And these same people were by now spending billions on CAM solutions.

Beginning as early as the 1970s, attempts to combine all these insights into an integrative—or, more recently, what is called an *integral* model of health care—have resulted in the creation of a new paradigm of medicine that is destined to both transcend and include the old reductionistic model. The ultimate triumph of the new medicine is only a matter of time.

I had tracked the alternative medicine movement for years, but I entered this stream with both feet around 1992, spurred on by the spectacular recovery of my wife and my desire to serve patients more effectively. But the watershed event for me was a meeting with a group of ten integrative medicine pioneers at the invitation of Russell Jaffe, the pioneering orthomolecular physician and researcher who had helped me to solve Vicki's illness. This seminal group—including five MDs, the owner of a nutraceutical firm, and several other health care professionals—met in 1992 at a San Francisco hotel for a one-day conference.

At this summit of like-minded colleagues, we took it as our initial task to coin a name for the new medicine. We felt that this name, along with a succinct definition, would help the broad "alternative" movement to become more easily institutionalized in clinical settings. What was needed was a designation that would express the essence of the emerging model, which was, at a minimum, holistic, patient-centered, and focused on wellness and prevention. It therefore seemed to us that terms like *natural medicine* and *holistic medicine* weren't quite satisfactory. A big part of the new model, of course, was the shift from disease care to a new vision of care oriented toward wellness and peak health. So the consensus was that the word *health* should be part of the new name. We then added the word *medicine* to stand for our openness to *all* healing disciplines that humanity has evolved throughout the millennia. Thus, the term *Health Medicine* was coined in a single, and for us historic, day.

This new phrase and its underlying concepts have grown and flowered ever since, especially in the San Francisco Bay Area. In fact, my own more recent experience has led me to a new level of understanding: I have added the term *integral* to the phrase, and I now call our movement *integral-health medicine*. But the model has been known as simply *Health Medicine* for most of its history.

Groping for an institutional model for Health Medicine

Soon after the San Francisco meeting, I gathered up my courage and made my first attempt to build an integrative medical center based on the Health Medicine concept. I had long been networking with open-minded colleagues in the region and had developed contacts with more than 50 health care practitioners, and it was time to act! So I convened an initial meeting, inviting them all—thereupon stumbling onto the first of many lessons in what it takes to establish a new institutional model of any sort, let alone one in corporate-dominated medicine.

Large-scale discussions proceeded over a period of months. It became clear to the group that an integrative-health center should provide one-stop shopping for health care services. The convenience of having many different disciplines under one roof would especially attract people interested in CAM, we thought. The resulting synergies would also create new business for each practitioner.

Attracting more business was on everyone's mind, and for a good reason. Insurance companies do not reimburse most CAM services—no matter how well evidenced and understood—and especially did not back then. For this reason, CAM practices tend to be small and insular, and practitioners are often reluctant to refer their patients to other practitioners for fear of losing them. But sharing them in an integrative center, we believed, might foster reciprocal referrals, allowing all of us to grow together as we better served our patients.

As we examined this concern and many related issues, it soon became clear that we had a great deal more to learn about the business and politics of organizing an integrative practice. First, dealing with the existing health care monopolies would be a big problem: We would be operating against the grain of conservative insurance companies, entrenched HMO medicine, hostile medical boards, and unfavorable laws. Plus, we were lacking in both experience and theory; we were pioneers with almost no existing, profitable models to draw lessons from. How would the center be organized? Would it be nonprofit or for-profit? How much money would be needed for the start-up, and from whom? How would we apportion the shared overhead? On what basis would we share our patients? How would we coordinate treatment programs among so many practitioners of diverse healing modalities?

We obviously needed expertise we did not have.

Other attempts to build such centers in those days were isolated cases, and many failed. As a result, there were no seasoned business consultants around to assist us—other than a courageous, growing coterie of researchers, visionaries, and academics, most of whom had little clinical experience and not much business sense. At the same time, we knew that the market demand was out there. But how would we package our services for these patients within a sustainable business model?

Most of the experiments up to this point had been idiosyncratic or not comprehensive enough to be truly integrative. It was only later, for example, that I learned about the pioneering work of John Travis, MD, who opened the country's first *wellness center* in 1975 nearby in Mill Valley, California.[1] It had focused almost entirely on educating people about wellness and prevention. Other features of an integrative clinic had been attempted elsewhere, but little was known about how to put these pieces together in a collaborative treatment methodology. Most of the early so-called integrative medicine clinics that succeeded financially did so because they were more a co-op of practitioners working in the same location but in separate offices, operating primarily as independent practitioners with their own private patients.

Of course, we had only tepid support from government—that is, when it was not actively resisting the free development of CAM and the integrative approach. Yet, some in Washington were getting the message. Almost concurrently with our local effort, the National Office of Alternative and Complementary Medicine was launched at the NIH in October 1991 with token funding of $2 million for fiscal year 1992. It was renamed the National Center for Complementary and Alternative Medicine (NCCAM) in October 1998. (NCCAM is now one of the 27 institutes and centers that make up the NIH at the U.S. Department of Health and Human Services.)

NCCAM was a step in the right direction, but even 11 years into its existence, controversy continues about whether or not its funding is being used to support or actually undermine CAM's development. CAM practitioners often find it very difficult to obtain funding for qualified research studies. Many of us believe the center is managed by researchers and bureaucrats committed to the allopathic paradigm, who are either approving studies likely to show that CAM does not work or directing its funds to more mainstream research studies. For example, a large percentage of the NCCAM budget (27 percent) in 2005–7 was spent on researching herbs, yielding data that could be exploited by pharmaceutical companies.[2]

There isn't much to fight over, in any case. Congress has given only token support for CAM to the NCCAM; its budget had risen to only $121 million in 2008, or much less than 1 percent of the NIH's $30 billion budget—and far less, for example, than the $195 million ad campaign that launched the destructive drug Vioxx!

The Health Medicine Forum is born

Now realizing what a formidable challenge we faced, in October 1994 I invited a group of six leading practitioners to meet at my home to start the discussion anew. Included in this new group were practitioners from Chinese medicine, chiropractic, bodywork, homeopathy, and psychology, and myself in internal medicine. This time, the discussion was more practical: We looked at issues such as insurance reimbursement, integrative treatment methodology, marketing tactics, barriers to collaboration, and the general difficulty of maintaining an independent practice in an HMO world. I made sure that we especially focused on how to work together for the benefit of our patients.

As destiny would have it, our immediate efforts *would not* lead to the creation of an integrative clinical center. The business issues we faced were huge and the politics were formidable. We thought it best to stay free-form and in learning mode, yet keep our intention firm. We were doing *paradigm work*. If we created an open space of gestation, a place of inquiry free of commercial pressure, perhaps an institutional manifestation would evolve from within this matrix. This made sense, and we soon found ourselves hosting and conducting a regular discussion forum. Within a few months after this small group's initial meeting, interest rapidly mounted, so we threw it open to health care practitioners from all disciplines in the San Francisco Bay Area.

As more people heard about our open forums for practitioners, our group meetings quickly grew to as many as 100 people. It wasn't long before we chose the name *Health Medicine Forum* (HMF) and began to formalize an organization. Our ambitious reason for forming the HMF was to reinvent how health care is practiced in America. That's still our goal.[3]

January 1995 was set as the formal launch date of the HMF, or the Forum, as this group is now affectionately referred to. At first we gathered to discuss what troubled us about medicine as it was then practiced. As we got to know one another, we learned what each of us did in our particular mainstream or CAM specialty—and there were many of them! As a group of committed professionals, we inquired rigorously into how each discipline works. In these early days, the focus of most meetings was on a "show and tell" agenda. Practitioners gave demonstrations so that everyone could see or experience firsthand a particular modality from the standpoint of the caregiver or the patient.

Interest in the Forum grew so quickly that within 18 months we found ourselves sponsoring a three-day symposium, which attracted 200 practitioners from a wide range of disciplines. We provided each professional with the opportunity to explain his healing modality, and we encouraged each one to explore with the entire conference how his approach might become part of a collaborative and integrative treatment approach. The symposium also considered the crucial distinction between curing and healing, and explored the difference between treating diseases and addressing the needs of the whole person. Many attendees spoke of the role of spirit in health and, ultimately, the healing power of love. The presentations were interspersed with singing and skits, and even included chanting, rituals, and prayer. Spirits were high, and the entire conference rocked with excitement.

The inspiring success of this conference led to yet another large event the following year, in 1998. This one featured many nationally known speakers and authors eager to participate in the growing Health Medicine movement. Our keynote speakers included Jerry Brown, Barry Sears, John McDougall, Jean Shinoda Bolen, Martin Rossman, Meg Jordan, Beverly Rubik, and many others. While the enthusiasm was high, at least one crucial ingredient was still missing: the practical wisdom and business acumen needed to bring Health Medicine into clinical practice.

The evolution of the Health Medicine model naturally unfolded from there. Gradually, the primary emphasis shifted to exploring real cases and experimenting with how specific disciplines might work together to create better health care for our patients. We termed these various combinations *multidisciplinary assessment and treatment teams*. Emerging from these experiments, the HMF developed a style that puts a patient in a circle with experts from varied disciplines. This was the origin of the *Health Medicine Healing Circle*, perhaps the most important innovation of the movement. We'll return to the subject of Healing Circles in the next chapter, as we examine how I have used Circles at my own integrative clinic.

Since the HMF's inception, more than 6,000 health care practitioners representing countless disciplines have attended at least one meeting there. As of this writing, the Forum has sponsored more than 350 meetings, workshops, and symposiums. Today our general meetings engage in interdisciplinary exploration of health care issues as these are related to diseases, treatment, research, economics, business, politics, and philosophy. Recent topics explored in the monthly symposiums have included sports medicine, energy medicine, holistic health testing, insomnia, diabetes, depression, integrative cancer strategies, and bodywork methods. We have reviewed these topics from the perspective of as few as one and up to as many as eight different disciplines in a single meeting. For example, when heart disease was the subject of one of our recent meetings, practitioners representing cardiology, psychology, biofeedback, Chinese medicine, Ayurveda, nutritional medicine, and Qi Gong were included. It is remarkable that most of the time, these widely differing styles of practice come to rather similar conclusions with regard to both diagnosis and treatment, despite the language and conceptual differences.

For 15 years, the HMF has continued to meet to define what Health Medicine is and how it should work. Among our achievements was the creation and refinement of a clinical model that embraces *four core Health Medicine principles*, as elucidated below. We've tested this model first on ourselves, and then on patients in pilot studies. Some of us have brought it into clinical practice. At least one enduring integrative clinic, my own, has arisen from this creative milieu of open-minded practitioners.

The evolution of the core principles of Health Medicine

Contrary to the expectations of skeptics, the HMF discovered in its experiments that most disciplines *can* work together with remarkable compatibility. This was perhaps our first major discovery. Conventionally trained physicians are at first wary of integrative approaches because they rightly fear that they will not be able to predict the net effect of a given combination of modalities. However, as I and others at the HMF began to build upon the early experiments and started to operate in at least rudimentary integrative settings, we found it uncommon that treatments indicated by one discipline interfered with those of another. *Indeed, not only were individual treatments comparable or even similar in outcome, but when several were simultaneously applied, the results were typically superior.* Put another way, each practitioner has a different perspective and uses unique tools, but together they can contribute to a higher, synergistic understanding of most diseases and of how to restore and maintain wellness.

We are still early on the learning curve. But as all of us in this field improve our treatment methodologies, we'll be able to maximize interdisciplinary synergies, minimize adverse effects, and anticipate where unexpected problems may develop. Assuming we can find ways to improve insurance coverage for integrative care, progress will also depend on good management practice, inspired integrative teamwork—and, as we'll see shortly, the further development of the integral theory of medicine.

Now, it must be admitted that adding a new treatment strategy to a given situation might bring new and unanticipated complications at times. But let's face it—that's what a large portion of the American population is already doing. We've noted that many patients have long been tossing together, ad hoc, various treatment modalities on their own—often secretly and for the most part unsupervised and uncoordinated. That's why, rather than having patients stealthily self-manage their ad-hoc integrative treatment regime, it is far better for everything to be out in the open and scrutinized in a genuinely integrative, professional setting. Unfortunately, this sort of scrutiny lags far behind the market demand for it.

Over time, the Forum came to agreement about our main beliefs. Aside from our intensive work with the integrative method, other common concerns arose and converged in a grand consensus. These included the imperative of lifestyle management and prevention, and the need to consider the whole person in our model of medicine. Today, the Forum's mission statement defines us as "a gathering of health-care practitioners committed to practice integrative, holistic, person-centered care that emphasizes wellness and prevention as primary strategies to support and maintain good health." Thus, the cornerstones of Health Medicine, though still evolving, now comprise the following four principles:

- Integrative practice

- Holism

- Person-centered care

- Prevention and wellness

Let's take a careful look at each one.

Integrative practice:
the first core principle of Health Medicine

A desire to work together as teams of healers was the driving force that originally brought most members of the Health Medicine Forum together. Our common objective has been to help patients in any way possible by being willing to consider all healing resources as potential options. If the goal of health care is to heal the sick and assist healthy people in maintaining their wellness, why exclude any options that might be helpful? Prejudice, arrogance, and sheer ignorance about how a particular discipline works are not acceptable reasons for exclusion.

I emphasize again that we are facing an epidemic of chronic diseases amid a general health-care delivery crisis. No single discipline or perspective has come anywhere near cracking the code of these diseases, not to mention many other health issues. *Every discipline can use all the help it can get.* Working in teams in which each practitioner brings her best health care strategies to the healing arena offers more than any single discipline could provide by itself. To me, this is so obvious that it defies logic to think that a more restrictive approach should have primacy.

During our first few months of exploration at the Forum, we began to appreciate the profound and complementary contributions of Native American medicine, Ayurveda, Chinese medicine, homeopathy, chiropractic, bodywork, guided imagery, and energy medicine. Of course, these and many other health care styles are often regarded by the mainstream as unscientific and therefore not reasonable to use—thus not reimbursable. Yet those who favor exclusion have usually done almost no homework. Nor do they sufficiently support objective research into the "new" modalities or comparative research across modalities or paradigms. So who's being unscientific?

The entire population of this planet has survived over millennia through the use of traditional and indigenous medical remedies—and 80 percent of the world's people still do. These practitioners learned from generations of practical experience about how to treat *whole persons.* They developed natural treatments in the context of cosmological worldviews worked out over centuries by the leading minds of their races or nations. Yet the budget for researching this vast store of healing wisdom is a tiny sliver of the NIH's overall annual budget, as we've seen. While one can readily admit that the cross-cultural comparison of medical treatments requires considerable research, we *do* have the resources to carry out this work if the willingness is there. For the sake of our patients, we need to take advantage of the present opportunity to harvest this hard-won practical wisdom and blend it into diverse sets of treatment strategies that are far more encompassing.

On the other hand, caution and discretion are also wise in these matters. My long clinical experience shows that a blend of disciplines is certainly not *always* the best approach. The art of the practice of integrative medicine entails knowing when mainstream medicine *alone* is clearly the best approach, while also being able to identify those times when a single CAM approach is superior. Of course, in most cases, a blend of several approaches or a progression of treatments is most advantageous.

In chapter 4, we noted that the optimal treatment methodology from the standpoint of cost containment requires the least invasive therapy to be undertaken first. For our current consideration, this hierarchy of treatment modalities bears repeating:

- Lifestyle strategies such as a healthy diet, adequate sleep and exercise, stress reduction, weight control, avoidance of toxic exposures, and securing emotional and spiritual balance in life are the *first line of defense.*

- Noninvasive complementary and alternative services such as acupuncture, herbal medicine, chiropractic, bodywork, homeopathy, and energy medicine are *the next line of defense.*

- Natural-medicine approaches based on the latest biomedical advances in orthomolecular medicine, functional medicine, and bioenergetic research—and including advanced forms of testing—are a *further line of defense.*

- Very careful and sparing use of pharmaceutical drugs, surgery, and other invasive strategies are *the last line of defense.*

Sometimes, the patient has progressed all the way to the point that the last line of defense is clearly indicated. A truly integrative methodology based on this hierarchy will ensure that this occurs.

Having access to a broad-based, carefully managed, integrative setting gives doctors and patients a larger repertoire of options and the freedom to choose what works. An integrative clinical setting also creates a context that can prevent a form of tragic dogmatism one sees all too often in patients—what you might call the "reverse dogmatism" of the rebel. This mentality rebels against the reductionist medical model by simply *inverting* it. Not unlike their alleged foes in disease care medicine, such patients will insist on limiting their treatment program to just *one particular* approach (in this case, some CAM modality of their choice), to the exclusion of anything else. When that fails, they will attach themselves to another CAM therapy. This especially seems to happen in cases of cancer, as illustrated in the examples below.

"JW" was in her mid 70s when she was found to have a very small breast cancer that could have easily been removed and would most likely have been cured by doing a simple lumpectomy.

I pleaded with her to have the lump removed surgically. But she was adamant that this was not necessary and that she could heal the cancer herself using CAM treatments exclusively. JW underwent almost every CAM therapy you could imagine. And she died seven years later with a large, foul-smelling, necrotic cancerous mass that had gradually spread to the rest of her body.

Another patient of mine who had a breast cancer that was a bit larger and more advanced did agree to have a lumpectomy. Her cancer was tested and found to be sensitive to estrogen. This was significant, because it is known that by blocking the effects of estrogen with mainstream hormonal therapies, it might be possible to slow the growth or spread of the tumor and extend life significantly. She adamantly refused this treatment because it was "too Western." About two years later, an enlarged lymph node was found in her axilla (the armpit area) that turned out to be cancerous. She again refused antiestrogen therapy and elected to try a variety of CAM anticancer treatments, flying overseas to the finest cancer treatment centers in Switzerland and Germany. Nothing worked, and the cancer spread to her lungs. I again suggested that she consider using the standard conventional treatment, but there was no way she'd have any part of it—she'd rather die than change her belief system. Seeing no choice, I supported the strategies in which she had faith. Even when she was terminal, there was still a good chance that the mainstream hormonal treatment would have helped. But no way was she going to "give in" to conventional therapy. She died a few weeks later in respiratory failure from the cancer.

On the flip side of this, another patient of mine had an enormous ovarian cancer. Over a couple of years, it filled her entire abdominal cavity, causing her to look about six months pregnant. Finally, she agreed to surgery, but mostly because the tumor's size was uncomfortable. The bulk of the tumor was removed, but remnants were scattered throughout her abdomen. Chemotherapy was now indicated, but she refused it; deep inside she knew that she would be OK. Her attitude was totally positive, and she was convinced beyond a shadow of doubt that she would beat the cancer from this point forward using healthy lifestyle strategies. It has now been about year and there's no evidence of any tumor growth. Go figure.

In another telling example of why we should all try to avoid reverse dogmatism, a chiropractor who had a terminal lymphoma showed up in my office one day. He came to me because he was totally opposed to chemotherapy or radiation and he thought I might be his last hope for some type of miracle CAM therapy. His weight had dropped from his usual 250 pounds to about 130 pounds. This man had palpable lymph nodes scattered all over his body, and he looked like death warmed over. I suspected he would live perhaps a few weeks longer if he continued on his course without conventional treatment. My advice was that he contact an oncologist for chemotherapy as soon as possible. Happily, he accepted my advice. Twelve years later, he's back to his normal weight and is living a full life practicing chiropractic and enjoying his kids and grandkids.

A professional colleague shared another, more mysterious cancer case. He had agreed to provide terminal care as a favor to a family friend. As part of his general supportive treatment, he gave this patient large doses of vitamin D_3, though he had no intentions of curing the cancer with the vitamin. Yet, within a few weeks, the tumors totally disappeared and the patient recovered!

As we evolve the new model of medicine, we must not become overconfident. Even with the expansion that comes with blending all possible perspectives on disease and wellness, we still don't know all the answers—especially with regard to complex maladies like cancer. Mainstream physicians often accuse CAM practitioners of malpractice when they do not advocate mainstream treatments and instead use approaches that have not been widely researched in clinical trials—and most states have laws that prohibit CAM treatments for cancer. CAM practitioners remind many mainstream oncologists who are quick to recommend invasive treatments that when it comes to treating themselves or their families, these oncologists are far more reluctant to use such treatments. So how does one get optimal cancer treatment? There is so much more to learn.

The pursuit of the integration of multiple disciplines is developing slowly. Today's medical school training strongly supports ongoing dialogue among the different fields within conventional medicine, but it does little to encourage dialogue between mainstream and CAM disciplines. By all accounts, the impetus to bring CAM into mainstream medical school training is coming from the students themselves and rarely from the faculty.

Again, a self-righteous attitude is not unique to mainstream physicians; it is also common in many CAM health care disciplines and their adherents. Much more work is needed, in theory, in clinical practice, and in business-model innovation, to advance the standard of integrative care beyond the current season of fragmentation.

The crucial contribution of integral theory, which is leading to the slow evolution of the integral-health medicine model— the true future of medicine—is broached in this chapter and in the final chapters of this book. The groundbreaking anthology *Consciousness and Healing*, by Marilyn Schlitz, Tina Amorok, and Marc Micozzi, offers a clarion call for the construction of this new, integrally informed paradigm of medicine.[4]

Holism (and integralism): the second core principle of Health Medicine

When we get sick, our illness affects us physically, mentally, emotionally, and spiritually; that's because body, mind, emotion, and spirit are *inseparably* interconnected. We are one and whole—not four detachable pieces like some jigsaw puzzle.

Consider, for example, the apple. The apple is just one thing: an apple. Yet, when seen from multiple points of view, it has different parts. It has a skin for protection, interior fruity substance, and seeds for replication, and it is made of billions of cells. It is grown by some agribusiness in pesticide-laden soil or on an organic farm; it goes into an apple pie or into a box lunch. Everything we can describe about the apple is part of the whole apple. Everything!

In the same way, each of us is a *single* human being. Any given part of us can be analyzed somewhat independently of all other parts, but we still remain one, unified entity. Of course, humans have many more ingredients than apples do: In addition to our exterior bodily existence and its many parts, made up of trillions of cells, we have an active *interior* life made up of *its* "parts," including thoughts, emotions, and spiritual impulses that are growing through many stages into maturity. Still, none of these elements can be separated from the whole person without destroying what we are, any more than we could separate the simple parts of an apple without destroying the apple.

We humans are a multifaceted whole, comprising a rich, bubbling interior life that is dynamically unified with an ultracomplex exterior body. We're hard-wired to respond to every experience we have in *all* of these domains—every single time. Every experience we will ever have in our lives has physical, mental, emotional, and spiritual components—whether we know it or not, and whether we understand them or not.

But the new advances in the integral theory of medicine teach us to include even *more* in our concept of the whole, experiencing person.

In addition to the interior (mind-heart-spirit) and exterior (bodily existence, including our brain and nervous system) of the individual, we must, as with our humble apple, also consider the influence of both the interior and exterior of the *collective life of the society* in which an individual is embedded. Our collective interior is constituted by the spiritual/religious or cultural belief systems that condition our individual choices, including health decisions; our collective exterior is the objective or external social, economic, political, and environmental systems (including air, food, water, and soil) in which we move in daily life.

Understanding all of this is crucial if one is to truly comprehend the whole person. Health practitioners of the future will view the patient through each of these windows, allowing them more options for prevention, curing, and healing.

While we are generally satisfied if we can get rid of our physical symptoms when we are ill, we also intuit that there is far more to restoring overall health. As we begin to revise and update the meaning of holism in terms of the new findings of integral theory, integral-health medicine practitioners will look beyond physical disability and psychological challenges, once these are understood, to address the root causes of illness by exploring the meaning of illness in the context of each patient's whole life story and how it relates to her society and the universe. Unless these dimensions of the underlying causes of illness are addressed, new symptoms might always emerge.

Physicians are generally very good at collecting information when they take a patient's medical history, do a complete physical examination, and order laboratory testing. They are usually excellent at determining what disease a person has. However, our deeper psychospiritual needs, and the role in our health of our sociocultural conditioning and environmental impacts far beyond the individual, are often revealed only through very sensitive and active listening, deep personal caring, excellent documentation, and probing and testing the patient at all levels. This process of assessment and treatment cannot be rushed. It takes time, more time than physicians have in today's managed care system. Even so, the ideal of total patient care must not be abandoned. We must find a way to provide holistic care to everyone.

One great ray of hope is the relatively new field of psychoneuroimmunology, which regards all facets of who we are to be in constant communication with one another; they work as a single unit, not two or several. Pioneers such as Candice Pert, author of the book *Molecules of Emotion*, and Martin Rossman, MD, author of *Fighting Cancer from Within*, describe how profoundly our thoughts, biochemistry, and physiology are interrelated and how powerfully they impact our health.[5]

Our thoughts are potent in ways that we greatly underestimate. Thoughts are made of real energy. Perhaps the realm of quantum biology may one day help explain how thoughts form, how they are transmitted, what effects they have—indeed, what they really *are*. We do know that within microseconds, our thoughts affect the internal biochemistry of the entire body, cause changes in our physiology, and affect how we feel. Social and cultural theory and research are also revealing how the *noosphere* of the collective mind of humanity influences our thoughts moment by moment, which in turn affect our health and well-being.

Other fascinating and extremely valuable health care disciplines—some ancient and some decidedly modern—are based on the premise that body, mind, emotion, and spirit are *one*. All of our experiences in each of these domains are stored consciously and unconsciously, and collectively they play important roles in how we think, feel, breathe, move, and act. These patterns persist long after the conscious mind has forgotten or repressed the original experience. They become ingrained in who we are and profoundly affects our behavior.

We can access these deep-seated memories and complexes in several interesting ways. At times this emergence can seem spontaneous, but they can be accessed more reliably through a wide range of approaches such as psychotherapy, hypnotherapy, imagery, meditation, bodywork, prayer, and chanting.

Consider the modality of bodywork. An experienced, well-trained practitioner can detect holding patterns in our muscles, breathing patterns, and movement, and can carefully guide a patient through the process of remembering how these holding patterns formed and how they can be released. In the words of the legendary physical therapist and bodyworker Marion

Rosen, "The body never lies . . . it may reveal what the mind wants most desperately to hide."

When tense areas are released through specialized forms of massage, long-forgotten experiences may surge into conscious awareness, hopefully at a time later in life when the patient is better equipped to resolve them. The automatic nature of our posture, breathing, and movement reveals powerful clues that can help us delve into the inner meaning of each of these patterns. The "felt" meaning of emotional traumas may be stirred up and reexperienced during Rosen bodywork sessions, just as they can from a variety of other bodywork styles, such as Rolfing, the Alexander Technique, and the Feldenkrais Method. "Getting out of our heads" and into a deeply experiential state can give us the opportunity to face emotional issues that we could not deal with when they originally occurred. Many issues that were challenging decades ago, especially those in early childhood, may not be so challenging when we're much older and have had the chance to grow wiser. Marion teaches that "[l]earning to be who we are, and not who we think we should be, underlies much of this aspect of bodywork."

While this style of work is not in itself "formal" psychotherapy, it nonetheless is a powerful tool. As you might imagine, an ideal situation would be for a bodyworker and psychologist to work together—one to bring up issues and the other to process them safely and effectively. The new field called *transpersonal bodywork* or *somatic psychotherapy* supports this approach.

I single out this example to illustrate just one of dozens of collaborations that are possible once an integral model of Health Medicine is embraced.

Person-centered care:
the third core principle of Health Medicine

As author John Robbins has so aptly written in his book *Reclaiming Our Health*, Americans are taking back the power they have given the medical profession to make health care decisions.[6] To begin with, only we can make certain choices in life. Our physicians cannot make us eat healthy food, exercise daily, sleep eight hours a night, control our stress levels, keep our weight down, and have a meaningful purpose in life. They could serve as lifestyle coaches, but generally they don't; they are busy writing prescriptions in an effort to correct what goes wrong when we don't take responsibility for caring for ourselves.

In addition, a healing relationship emerges when both patient and healer cocreate a plan to transform the patient's situation from disease to wellness. As one of my mentors, Richard Miles, so eloquently points out, the healer's role is to "be with" rather than to just "do to" patients. As he so succinctly puts it, "Healing is much more than treating a set of symptoms with a bag of tools." Instead of this conventional "curing" approach, Richard feels that therapies should be offered to patients on the basis of whether they are congruent with the patients' preferences and belief system. This requires a willingness to listen to what patients are requesting, with an open mind and without bias or conflict of interest. It means that practitioners must not be overly invested in their own economics or the biases of their particular training; they must be willing to educate, but also be able to respect the choices that patients make and support their efforts to achieve them.

Of course, this does not happen most of the time. Practitioners from all disciplines tend to pressure their patients to deal with their health care issues based on the nature of their own particular training and *their* personal belief system—that is, unless they have expanded their minds and hearts through the embrace of an integrative methodology. If faced with rigid practitioners in a closed-loop institutional setting, patients often make end runs around them, as we've noted, subverting their own treatment program by covertly visiting alternative practitioners and adding different therapies.

Again, all of this will be out in the open when the patient is being seen in a genuine integrative setting. Healing options can then be fully discussed and uniquely tailored to each person's personality type and deeply held values. Experienced practitioners know that advice patients *believe in* is far more likely to be followed than advice they do not understand, do not have confidence in, or simply do not want to follow. Believing in one's treatment is far more likely to lead to what we conventionally call *patient compliance*—and as we'll see in the next section, it opens up the possibility of unleashing innate self-healing powers.

Person-centered care: the beliefs of the patient and the placebo effect

Medical science has repeatedly documented that our thoughts and emotions have a powerful effect on both causing and healing disease. Most of us are familiar with the concept of psychosomatic illness—that our bodies react to our thoughts and emotions in a way that leads to physical *dis-ease*. We know that stress can result in a myriad of diseases ranging from headaches to ulcers. We also know, perhaps even more important, that too much stress aggravates all diseases because it eventually wears us down and impairs our immunity. The importance of having a health care practitioner who understands this premise and who will take time to deal with the underlying causes of the patient's stress cannot be overemphasized. When this is done, the influence of the patient's core beliefs on medical outcomes often becomes paramount.

It is extremely odd that in mainstream medicine, health benefits that can be ascribed only to the effects of our belief system—resulting from the *placebo effect*—are presumed to be of no "real" value. Placebo therapy is generally regarded as out of bounds in medical practice. It is thought to be unethical to prescribe a sugar pill or a sham technology under the guise that it is a pharmacologically active drug or proven technology. Notably, in many forms of indigenous healing, this essential therapy is often used as powerful medicine.

Nevertheless, many doctors subvert the party line in practice; they seem to understand placebo power intuitively. In a study published in the January 2008 issue of the *Journal of General Internal Medicine*, the authors sent questionnaires to 466 internists at the University of Chicago inquiring about the use of placebos in their practices. Forty-five percent of the 231 who responded reported that they had used a placebo at some time in their clinical practice.[7] Only 12 percent responded that placebo use should be categorically prohibited. A growing number of physicians believe in the mind–body connection and are using it in their practices.

Yet most scientific studies published in major medical journals factor out the placebo effect when measuring the effect of a drug or technology. This may be valid as far as assessing the independent effects of a drug or technology, but is it good science to ignore a genuine healing phenomenon that is safe, affordable, and effective—simply because it is provided solely through the power of the human mind? In her fascinating study of our innate power of self-healing, *Faith and the Placebo Effect*, Lolette Kuby proclaimed, "If it is true that in every way placebos mimic 'active' drugs and intentional treatments, isn't it reasonable to ask whether the placebo produces a drug effect, or a drug produces a placebo effect? Instead of controlling to eliminate the placebo, I should think that medical experiments would attempt to reproduce it."

Our practice of ignoring the placebo effect, she points out, may be the result of commercial influence on how medical science is practiced. Limiting attention to the direct effect of a drug or technology obviously favors the sale of drugs and technologies; it eliminates any competition from the pluralistic worldview of our most powerful integrative healers—who may want to rely, as the occasion demands, on high-tech or noninvasive approaches, including placebo, depending on the patient's needs.[8]

Ask yourself: Do you prefer a therapy that is expensive, has side effects that can kill, and *still* may not work, or do you prefer one that has no side effects, costs nothing, and accounts for about 50 percent of the action of most drugs and technologies? For many situations this seems like a no-brainer! Yet we have been brainwashed by people touting scientific purity into believing just the opposite.

To illustrate this issue, let's take a close look at the commonly used class of drugs known as SSRI antidepressants. Among them is Prozac, still the most popular, with over 20 million prescriptions written in 2007 for its generic formulation. The early "scientific" studies of Prozac in the 1980s were mostly supported by the pharmaceutical industry. They concluded that it relieved symptoms of depression 59 percent of the time, whereas the placebo worked only 28 percent of the time. Therefore, it was deemed appropriate to use Prozac rather than the placebo. At the time, expected side effects of the drug were thought to be "minimal," but we now know that this is simply untrue. The lengthy profile of Prozac provided by its manufacturer in the *Physicians' Desk Reference* describes its pluses and minuses, mostly minuses. The list of possible problems is extensive. One recent study found that postmenopausal women taking SSRI antidepressants were twice as likely to suffer osteoporotic bone fractures.[9] Other studies show that SSRIs can induce suicidal thinking and even suicide, particularly in children.[10]

And how about the comparative effectiveness of SSRIs? In a revelation of the disease care mentality of some mainstream physicians, many prescribe antidepressants with their long list of potential dangerous side effects, even though moderate exercise—with its long list of positive side effects—turns out to be at least as effective. In *Archives of Internal Medicine* in October 1999, James Blumenthal and colleagues reported on their study out of Duke University comparing the effects of Zoloft (another SSRI antidepressant) and exercise in 156 people over 50.[11] People in the exercise group worked out for 30 minutes several times per week at about 75 percent of their maximum heart rate for 16 weeks. While both approaches worked equally effectively at reducing depressive symptoms, after six months 38 percent of those people on Zoloft had a return of their depressive symptoms, whereas only 8 percent of the exercise group relapsed. The authors found that "[f]or each 50-minute increment of exercise, there was an accompanying 50 percent reduction in relapse risk." It is clear that working out should be regarded as a major part of the treatment regime for depression, along with diet, sleep, and other lifestyle choices. It is equally clear that, on occasion, antidepressants are invaluable in temporarily clearing the symptoms of depression so that people can then function well enough to begin dealing with their emotional issues. However, antidepressants never, ever, ever, ever deal with the underlying issues that originally led to the depression. In my opinion, antidepressants are primarily a consideration for short-term usage.

In a more recent study, published in the August 2007 issue of *Psychosomatic Medicine*, Blumenthal's research team compared the effects of exercise, Zoloft, and placebo on 202 depressed patients.[12] After 16 weeks, they found that 47 percent of the patients on Zoloft, 45 percent of those doing only exercise, and 31 percent in the placebo group no longer met the criteria for major depression. It is interesting to speculate as to why Blumenthal did not test a fourth group with a combination of exercise and placebo. In any case, when you analyze the overall benefit of Zoloft over placebo in Blumenthal's study, it is remarkable that there was a mere 16 percent additional benefit for those patients taking Zoloft; but of course Zoloft has many, many more side effects than either a sugar pill or an exercise program.

More recent research darkens the picture considerably: It points to the possibility that *antidepressants actually work only marginally better than placebo.* In one probably definitive study, the six most widely used antidepressants scored just *two points higher* than placebo out of 62 possible points on the most widely used depression scale. According to the researchers, this meant that SSRI antidepressants are "very unlikely to be of any clinical importance."[13]

Could the inability to commercialize placebo therapy be the main reason why it is so often not used in clinical practice? How much money could be generated from the sale of a placebo? Could you imagine a pharmaceutical company supporting the use of a placebo instead of a drug that is making billions of dollars a year in sales? And what does all this mean for person-centered care?

Person-centered care: harvesting the lessons of illness

Even an illness as simple as a cold offers valuable insights. Perhaps we have gotten insufficient sleep, are under too much pressure at work, or have experienced too much physical stress. While each person's cold symptoms might be treated with similar medicines, their underlying causes are much more varied and may require more or less intensive investigation, depending on the particular person and her life situation.

We have repeatedly highlighted that the symptoms of illness are often the symbolic expression of much deeper issues; we humans tend to somatize our deeper psychospiritual problems. Sigmund Freud, Carl Jung, Wilhelm Reich, and their successors in the psychoanalytic tradition extensively explored this truth. And in relation to general health issues, such popular writers as Louise Hay, among many others, have written extensively on this topic for the layperson. Hay recounts amazing stories that often provide jarring insights into the possible deeper meaning of illness.

As a rule, then, the deeper meaning of illness is usually unconscious. Accessing these lessons requires a willingness to be more open and vulnerable if the deeper message is to be revealed. Most physicians are neither open to this work nor trained in such intuitive or analytical approaches to medical diagnosis and treatment.[14] But consider the fact that the word *physician* is derived from the Greek word for "teacher." Health Medicine encourages an educational, truth-seeking partnership between practitioner and patient wherein the practitioner is willing to be personally involved and vulnerable, just like the patient. This is, of course, a huge departure from my own training at Duke University, which emphasized "objective" detachment from patients.

When we are compromised by chronic illness, our need for supportive and loving human relationships becomes heightened. In this situation, we are often less able to care for our own needs and also less able to satisfy the needs of our friends and family. Unfortunately, fulfilling the needs of significant others may be a critical factor in maintaining these primary relationships. As a consequence, they may disintegrate when we need them the most. At times like this, our health care practitioners may be our only source of support.

Perhaps the most disastrous situations along this line—the direst examples of sufficient care not being directed to a patient's unique needs—occur when people are hospitalized and in critical condition. Far too often people die alone, without a family member, a friend, or even a health care professional at their side. Yet it is not realistic to expect practitioners who are out of touch with their *own* mortality to be able to support the deeper psychospiritual needs of the dying. Put simply, they cannot offer patients what they have not already achieved for themselves.

In fact, mainstream medical training cuts the other way. Young physicians are taught to favor an adversarial stance against nature and death, leading them to "fight to the end" to preserve life—often ignoring what the patient or the patient's family wants, and with little respect for the intrinsic nature of the life cycle or for the staggering expenses associated with the fight. When a doctor "loses" a patient, it is even equated to losing a battle in the war against nature.

By contrast, many ancient indigenous cultures viewed the life cycle as something natural, finite, and perfect. It was considered sacred. They believed that the passage from life as we know it on earth to another dimension deserves to be honored and celebrated. *Indeed, the passage to death itself can be a form of healing.* A key role of Health Medicine practitioners is to support dying patients by honoring their spiritual preferences and by being willing to be with them to provide the vital spiritual guidance they need until they pass on to another world. It is a time when there is often nothing "medical" to do; it is a time to be with them in a state of compassion, love, understanding, and support.

Prevention and wellness:
the fourth core principle of Health Medicine

As modern medicine became increasingly preoccupied with fighting disease as a business proposition, it all but forgot about wellness and prevention—the fourth and last principle developed by the Health Medicine Forum. The old saying "An ounce of prevention is worth a pound of cure" may sound a bit corny, but it is right on the mark when it comes to maintaining good health. And yet, less than 5 percent of the NIH budget is allocated to prevention and wellness![15]

The war on cancer has spent untold billions in a largely fruitless search for cures for various types of cancer, giving little serious attention to preventing this scourge. What about heart disease, the other great killer? Modern medicine provides ingenious treatments such as stents, surgeries, and drugs for people with arteriosclerotic heart disease, but it rarely addresses preventive lifestyle strategies—even though the science proves that these strategies are highly effective in preventing and even reversing the process that led to the disease in the first place.

A fascinating pilot study led by Dean Ornish, MD, published in 2008 in the *Proceedings of the National Academy of Sciences*, points to the great promise of prevention and lifestyle measures.[16] In this controlled experiment, men with low-grade prostate cancer were put on an intensive healthy diet and lifestyle regime emphasizing low meat and high vegetable and fruit intake, regular exercise, yoga, stretching, meditation, and support group participation. The study documented the fact that this *lifestyle alteration alone* had the power to change the progression of prostate cancer. It accomplished this feat by switching on tumor-killing DNA and turning down the tumor-promoting DNA in about 500 genes! Two very hopeful conclusions can be drawn from this finding: First, when combined with other findings in the emerging field of epigenetics, it overturns the idea that DNA structure is fixed and unchangeable. Second, it illustrates that *the power of lifestyle is finally becoming understood at the level of molecular biology.*

The time has indeed come to embrace wellness and prevention as *primary medicine* rather than as an afterthought. Toward this end, a group of well-known experts in the new field of preventive medicine—including Dean Ornish of UCSF, Walter Willett of Harvard Medical School, and many other internationally distinguished people—are just now coming together to lead an international movement that embraces lifestyle medicine. The American College of Lifestyle Medicine was formed in 2005 and has its own medical journal, the *American Journal of Lifestyle Medicine.*

But is lifestyle really at the root of cancer and heart disease? Remember that just 100 years ago, our two biggest killers were *uncommon diseases.* We certainly carry the genetic capacity for cancer and heart attacks, but their high incidence today can't possibly be attributed to a century of random genetic mutation. So why have they become epidemic diseases in such a short time—that is, as biological evolution measures time? What is different today compared with 100 years ago? The answers are simple. Going back to our previous model, there are only four pathways at the level of the cell that lead to illness: genetics, toxic exposures, nutritional deficiencies, and psychospiritual stresses.

The factors that have changed over the last hundred years are the latter three—profoundly so. Interestingly, the term *lifestyle* is inclusive of all three.

We've noted the dramatic changes in what we eat as we migrated from rural to urban life. After millennia of eating fresh, whole foods off the land, we now consume packaged food products that are refined, processed, and polluted with a wide range of insecticides, pesticides, food additives, and preservatives. As we noted earlier, we are only beginning to appreciate the far-reaching effects of the decreased nutritional density and increased pollution of our food. And this does not even factor in the known and unknown potential effects of genetically engineered, X-rayed, or microwaved foods, or foods containing trans fats or high-fructose corn syrup, or foods low in fiber.

We have also managed to pollute our food, water, air, and soil over the past century. More than 100,000 new chemicals have been synthesized and scattered over the planet. While we know the toxic effects on our bodies of many of these chemicals, we've barely touched the surface of what they can do in combinations. We have unwittingly conducted a global experiment on what happens when we poison ourselves!

Finally, our levels of psychospiritual stress have increased. Our technology has encouraged us to constantly stay on the fast track. We are suffering from an epidemic of working too long and too hard, getting too little sleep, spending too little time with our families and friends, eating too much, and forgetting that we're human beings on a spiritual path.

One must almost be deaf and blind not to appreciate what harm we've done to ourselves over the past century. Yet we've managed to ignore this tragic situation and have relied on the promises of our medical system to fight disease *after the fact* with drugs and technologies. Antibiotics, steroids, birth control pills, and even Viagra were celebrated as breakthroughs proving how man could triumph over nature through science. This power struggle has continued, and now we have an enormous arsenal of treatments designed to fight every symptom and disease known to man. While we have made some progress in helping people to feel better and enjoy healthier lives, this kind of thinking has nonetheless caused an ongoing epidemic of chronic diseases and has led to the soaring costs of today's health care.

Americans are awakening to this sad state of affairs. They want a major transformation in health care, and the Health Medicine movement and its core principles have arisen from the grassroots efforts of hundreds of practitioners to address their demands. To support this revolution, in chapter 9 we offer five specific measures that policymakers can implement to encourage prevention at all ages.

And yet, no matter how good prevention and wellness may sound, we cannot expect to switch from a disease care system to a true health care system without a major battle. Think of what might happen if we suddenly didn't need so many drugs, technologies, physicians, and hospitals, plus all the other supporting layers of the medical-industrial complex that now comprises 18 percent of the American economy. If a sane system of health care is to evolve in America, politicians and business leaders must seek compassionate methods for replacing the income and the enormous number of jobs that the obsolete disease care model now generates. Perhaps thousands of new jobs can be generated in the emerging prevention, wellness, CAM, and integrative medicine industries; from expansion of organic agriculture; and through single-payer health care insurance, which alone could generate over two million new jobs, according to projections of the Institute for Health and Socio-Economic Policy.[17]

It is time to take a hard look at this situation. It is not enough to make the paradigm shift from disease care to health care in our thinking; we must also explore how to ensure that the transition is economically feasible without a traumatic blow to our economy— even as we seek a practical clinical model based on the Health

Medicine revolution, the subject of the next chapter. We have no other choice but to pursue the resolutions of these issues if we are going to reduce the cost of a health care system that jeopardizes the solvency of our government and the very quality and length of our lives.

Eight

Creating an Integrative Medical Clinic

An "integral medical practice" is a practice that makes room
for the entire panoply of effective treatments.

−Ken Wilber

An integrative medicine approach seeks to discern multiple
perceived origins of a disease process and address them all.
Integrative medicine also assumes that an individual has
the potential for healing at the spiritual level, even when
physical healing does not take place.

−Andrew Weil, MD

The first integrative clinic based on Health Medicine was born almost literally amid the flames of a real fire. In September 2001, the building in which I was practicing medicine suddenly burned to the ground. This strangely timed conflagration had synchronicity written all over it. A fire had now been lit under me to create a center for health medicine. It was as if the old medicine had gone up in smoke, and the universe were shouting, "It's time to begin the work you've long dreamed about!"

It had been a long time coming. The Health Medicine Forum (HMF) had been founded in 1994 and spent seven years exploring how the principles of health medicine could be applied in clinical practice; it was high time to test the model that I had helped pioneer.

Within a few weeks, I secured an office that would become the new home for a clinical center, a research institute, and the meetings of the Forum itself. We named it the Health Medicine Institute (HMI). Waiting in the wings was an investor, Bob Leppo, and a CEO that Bob recruited, Kay Sandberg. They almost immediately came on board to help initiate the new venture. The three of us brought all the vision, management expertise, and capital needed to start up the ambitious project. We opened our doors by November 2001, less than two months after the fire!

HMI's founding practitioners included a bodyworker specializing in post-traumatic stress therapy, a Chinese medicine practitioner, a registered nurse with expertise in energy medicine, a psychologist, a naturopath, a chiropractor with side specialties in homeopathy and applied kinesiology, and myself, a board-certified physician in internal medicine. This diverse team soon found itself creating integrative health care solutions for many patients, notably those who had been going from doctor to doctor without much success.

Because this was such a novel experience for all of us, building camaraderie among our practitioners was a primary goal from the beginning. HMI sponsored retreats where we cooked, ate, worked, and played together. We explored visions of the new medicine, shared about our disciplines, and worked through the nuances of our personal and professional relationships with one another. Gradually, we evolved into a trusting family of healers that was able to collectively guide our patients through recovery.

One of our first patients was Jason. He came to HMI because he had heard about our photonic stimulation device and our integrative pain management program, which rarely uses medications to control pain (introduced in chapter 3). At age 32, he was considering suicide because of intense, unrelenting pain and the negative effects it was having on his marriage, employment, and quality of life. He had suffered through two failed back surgeries for lumbar disc problems that left him in constant pain despite the use of narcotics, antidepressants, anti-inflammatory drugs, and muscle relaxants. He had become a "walking zombie" who could not find any position where his pain would relent. He was on total disability, his marriage had crumbled, and pain and depression had become a way of life.

Our HMC team of practitioners met and created a collaborative plan of treatment, and I assumed the role of being Jason's *health guide*. His insurance was minimal, of course, so most of the care he received was gratis. I still wonder how much of his recovery was related to the fact that, out of compassion, we gave our time without concern about compensation.

Jason's initial treatment with the new photonic device in whose use we are pioneers provided his first break from pain in nearly four years. Within a few weeks of starting his full treatment program—which also included acupuncture, bodywork, chiropractic, and guided imagery—he was able to discontinue all medications. He began taking walks and could now sleep through the night without pain. He soon joined a gym and regained much of his lost muscle strength. Within a few months, Jason took up his interest in golf again, was looking for work, and had become socially active. Today, about eight years later, Jason visits us about once a month for a light treatment and a chiropractic adjustment. As he now puts it, "I have my life back!"

We soon learned that synergy is an essential part of the clinical practice of integrative medicine. Working in the same location, and often together at the same time, can be far more effective than coordinating care with practitioners in independent offices, which causes a patient's health care to be fractured into pieces managed by several specialist physicians or independent CAM practitioners.

Indeed, without the structured collaboration provided by an integrative clinic, the *patient* is forced to do the overall coordination! It can't be stated often enough: Long experience and simple logic show that integrative medicine under one roof is far superior to the fragmented care provided by either standard mainstream medicine or CAM therapies alone, or by diverse approaches blended in an ad hoc manner without professional coordination.

Over the course of our initial five years at HMI, we branched out even further in our integrative methodology. We attracted and worked with practitioners from a wide range of disciplines aside from our core group. Additional healing options beyond those mentioned above included Native American shamanism, Reiki, yoga, Qi Gong, marriage counseling, nutritional counseling, many styles of chiropractic, women's health, guided imagery, and movement therapies, as well as frontier technologies such as photonic stimulation, breast thermography, bioenergy testing, heart-rate variability testing, vascular stiffness testing, HeartMath, and dark field microscopy. A marvelous blend of what might be called high-tech and high-touch health care was evolving. And this was the beginning of the Healing Circles process that I have carefully developed over the years in collaboration with my colleagues, which I present later in this chapter.

Practical challenges in our first integrative clinic

As the patient load increased, I discovered what a joy it was to work in a team setting that had the capacity to treat the whole person. It had been a long time in the making, and it was working as well as we had hoped. But one problem deeply troubled all of us. While it was very satisfying to help people who could afford our services, there were far too many who could not. There were a few like Jason that we simply did not have the heart to turn away, but we also knew we could not afford to see the vast majority of people who couldn't pay for their care if we wanted to keep our doors open. We were running into the deep prejudice against CAM and the integrative model that to this day plagues government policy and the private health insurance business.

Eventually we ran into other problems—everyday business issues that will always afflict integrative health care clinics as long as we must operate against the grain of the current paradigm.

For example, we found it difficult to recruit CAM practitioners who already had full and successful practices. Put simply, they were reluctant to bring their clientele with them. Why should they? They were content with being in solo practice, where they could call their own shots while at the same time enjoying financial security. They were providing competent care, no doubt, but from our perspective they were also becoming entrenched as just another species of the fragmentation of health care delivery in a time of competing paradigms and poor government coordination. They too were not ready for the integrative model of the future. Plus, most were forced to operate among the affluent; they were occupying the finite market of those wealthier patients who could pay out of pocket.

On the other hand, for those CAM practitioners just starting out (or who perhaps were not as strong at marketing), things were different. Again, unfair discrimination against CAM by policymakers and insurance providers limits their reach in the market. Thus, unlike mainstream physicians, few CAM practitioners have full practices. Competition for patients can be fierce, leaving them with little incentive to refer patients to fellow CAM practitioners for fear of losing them and the income they generate. We consequently discovered an abundance of alternative practitioners looking primarily for work; they would work anywhere they could make an income. But they weren't motivated by a compelling interest in practicing collaborative Health Medicine.

In addition, although it was a responsibility of HMI practitioners to bring in patients and be willing to share them, many that we retained on staff were reluctant to recruit on behalf of the whole center. While a few were skilled at marketing, most were either unable or unwilling to build their practices in a collaborative way; they were far more comfortable waiting for patients to show up on their doorstep or come through referrals from within HMI. Competition for patients even *among* practitioners at HMI was a serious issue that did not lend itself to quality integrative health care. Several practitioners felt sufficiently insecure about their limited practice size that they left and took the patients they acquired while working at HMI. We just let them go; it was not worth bothering to enforce the noncompete clauses in their contracts.

But the biggest problem of all, as I have indicated, is that CAM services are largely nonreimbursable under the coverage rules of conventional health insurance companies. It can't be emphasized enough that this limits Health Medicine to those who can afford to pay for services in cash, thus collapsing the potential market. Even so, the CAM sector is still greater than the size of the out-of-pocket portion of the mainstream medical market, as noted earlier.

In any case, this insurance dilemma represents a serious inequity; it means that the playing field is not level between mainstream physicians and CAM practitioners. The mainstream enjoys a substantial competitive and strategic edge—even within Medicare and Medicaid—largely through the force of insider politics, the inertia of the health care system we have inherited, and the distraction of an unresolved conflict of paradigms.

This is a tragic situation for the American people. We HMC practitioners know from our experience that the integrative, holistic, preventive, and highly personalized model of Health Medicine is demonstrably more effective in solving even the most complex health care problems, and it is also clearly less expensive than mainstream health care. Yet, insurance companies—in the thrall of the monopolistic practices of the mainstream—dare not support integrative medicine wholeheartedly.

Some employers and insurance companies now offer FSAs—flexible savings accounts—allowing a certain number of dollars each year to be dedicated to any CAM service that the insured desires. Another version of this concept is the health savings account (HSA). These two approaches form the core of the emerging *consumer-directed* insurance plans, which impose greater cost-sharing on enrollees but permit some tax savings plus broader choices than the HMO plans of the managed care era. However, these approaches are underutilized and are beset with difficulties in practice.

We at HMI were up against an entrenched and at times hostile system, and before long, our seed money ran out. We simply could not attract enough people willing or able to pay out of pocket for enough of their health care, even in our affluent location. And we also had the kinds of operational problems that business pioneers always face. By October 2007 we were forced to close HMI's doors and reorganize our business plan.

Starting over again
with an improved clinical model

Undaunted, I immediately opened a new incarnation of HMI that was scaled down in size and ambition; I had learned to accept the fact that an integrative center will never be as profitable as any mainstream medical clinic as long as monopolistic forces are arrayed against us. We named it the Health Medicine Center (HMC), and it is still operating in Walnut Creek, California.[1]

The administrative and marketing aspects of HMC's business plan are substantially different from HMI's, yet the concept (of what I now call integral-health medicine) remains the same. We relocated from an upscale 5,000-square-foot building to one that is about 1,000 square feet. In this strategically designed smaller space, we are still able to accommodate 12 health care practitioners (who operate in shifts) and thus can still provide all the specialized tests and services that were offered at HMI.

In HMC's new model, practitioners are not expected to bring in new business; they primarily see patients who are referred from my internal medicine practice. As in the earlier model, the practitioners have continued to work together closely, meeting regularly to review treatment plans for our patients and conducting Healing Circles when needed. Cross-referrals often occur, and typically our patients will see several of us simultaneously.

We're continually evolving; even now we are examining the applicability of the new integral model of medicine to clinical practice. Overhead expenses for this operation are considerably lower than HMI's, but the quality and nature of care has not changed. HMC offers each practitioner a contract for services that include office space, support staff, appointment scheduling, and whatever other services are required to conduct each specific practitioner's business. The major difference between the HMI contract and HMC's is that we no longer require practitioners to build their practices; they are free to manage the size of their practice as they see fit. We have found that this updated model works well and believe it will be financially sound when the playing field is leveled; we further believe it has the potential for replication. However, we'll need to wait until that day when the insurance industry begins reimbursing for CAM services fairly.

Because of broad popular demand, there are a rapidly growing number of integrative health care clinics in the U.S. Most major medical facilities, such as large mainstream clinics, hospitals, and teaching centers, purport to offer CAM services. In general, however, they offer merely token services with limited, uncoordinated access to a few disciplines such as acupuncture, chiropractic, and massage—primarily window dressing designed to attract a larger market share of more enlightened consumers.

Healing Circles: a key innovation

The concept of Healing Circles evolved directly out of the Health Medicine movement, and has been fully explored by its pioneers at HMI and currently at HMC.

Patients best suited for Healing Circles are those with chronic diseases of such severity that they interfere with the patients' ability to enjoy healthy, functional lives. Typically, these patients have consulted numerous health care practitioners over periods of years; some have all but given up hope that recovery is possible. Many have traveled great distances or spent enormous sums of money trying a myriad of CAM therapies hoping to find a solution to their problem.

The Circles are composed of three to eight practitioners from a variety of disciplines, plus the patient. Everyone meets in a designated room, sitting together in a circle for approximately two hours. Before convening, the patient meets with a *health guide* for the purpose of determining which practitioners to invite. While it is preferable that the patient's primary care practitioner act as the health guide, outside practitioners with a broad knowledge of health care disciplines and CAM—such as a holistically oriented nurse or a broad-minded psychologist—can be trained to serve as the health guide.

Years of experience with Circles have shown that patients receive a number of benefits from them:

- First of all, patients usually receive immediately practical information in regard to resolving their illness from the point of view of several disciplines.

- Second, they often feel more empowered to delve into their psychospiritual problems—which are, after all, at the root of most diseases. In other words, patients receive excellent technical information offered from varied points of view, while also feeling supported to dive deeper into the meaning of their illness.

- But more important, perhaps, is that Circles usually witness a shift from information exchange to profound group interconnectedness. Powerful healing often emerges from the nature of the relationship between practitioners and the patient, and even from the practitioners' contact with one another. We have found that as each person becomes more authentic within a Circle, something like a descent into the soul occurs: All the connections deepen. This leads to a heightened awareness of the meaning of the illness in question and usually reveals the strategic approach most suitable in light of that deeper connection.

Practitioners who have participated in our Healing Circles include physicians of many mainstream disciplines, such as internists, psychiatrists, oncologists, family practitioners, neurologists, cardiologists, and surgeons. Complementary practitioners have included acupuncturists, chiropractors, herbalists, bodyworkers, homeopaths, nutritionists, naturopaths, Ayurvedic practitioners, indigenous healers, and many others. Although the composition of Healing Circles nearly always includes at least one conventional medical practitioner, it emphasizes the inclusion of all practitioners the patient has chosen to work with.

As integrative medicine becomes more mainstream and as the benefits of Healing Circles are better known, I believe that Circles will soon see participation from an even broader range of specialists and will involve into new forms and new applications, opening up even more options for healing for many patients.

How Healing Circles work in practice

Before participating in a Healing Circle, patients are asked to describe in writing why they are requesting a panel and what they hope to gain from the experience. They also are required to write an autobiography of their physical, emotional, and spiritual life since birth. Each panelist carefully reviews this information before the meeting convenes.

Our Circles always convene in a quiet, relaxing, and private setting. The health guide continues to take the lead, acting as moderator; the guide also concludes the session by providing a summary of each practitioner's input, including the recommended treatment strategies and goals.

After introductions, the process usually begins with the patient describing why he has requested a Circle, what his health issues are, and what he hopes to achieve. Practitioners are then encouraged to address their remarks directly to the patient whenever possible. Patients are assured that they are not expected to respond to questions that they feel are invasive.

In the Circle setting, health care professionals partner to support a single patient. The responsibility to help the patient is *shared* by all practitioners. This allows individual practitioners to feel less pressure to find a solution to the patient's problems. Not knowing becomes a more acceptable option, which permits the possibility for no action as an approach.

But does the decision for no action with a sick patient make sense? All too often, a one-on-one clinical setting carries with it the obligation to come up with a treatment, almost *any* treatment, so that at least "something" is seemingly being done. But in reality, not taking action can be far better than interventions that have little chance of helping, may give false hope, may be dangerous, or could lead to patient disappointment, frustration, anger, or even lawsuits. In fact, holding open the option for no action can be a blessing. It allows for a type of gentleness and wise forbearance not usually found in disease care medicine, with its invasive, know-it-all posture.

Once this kind of wisdom has been invoked, we have found that the best approach is to change the focus from curing to *healing*. In a Circle, this means supporting psychospiritual needs rather than forcing a treatment plan that has little chance of resolving what may be an impossible physical challenge. Happily, not much is required to carry out this subtler mission, since the group process of a Circle almost inevitably transforms itself from information exchange into heartfelt connection. In the right context, the human heart naturally shifts to regarding and treating the whole person rather than just curing disease or its symptoms.

Years of experience have shown us that the active and sensitive listening we practice in our Circles creates a sacred space in which patients feel deeply heard and cared for. While curing symptoms is still a high priority in most cases, Healing Circles also create a rich opportunity to explore the meaning of illness in the context of who the patient is—in relation to her entire life story, including her family, her culture, her lifework, and her total environment. In other words, they stimulate an *integral* approach to healing and evoke the entire spectrum of possibilities in the integral-health medicine model.

With the health guide still moderating, the practitioners hold a brief post–Healing Circle meeting without the patient. Its purpose is to review the group process, assess the strengths and weaknesses of the Circle, and receive full input from each practitioner for the final treatment plan, unless of course the no-action option has been chosen. The health guide writes a summary of the plan, sends it back to each practitioner for final edits, and then forwards it to the patient.

Each Healing Circle is unobtrusively recorded and transferred to a CD, with a copy stored for future reference. We recommend that patients listen to the CD as well as carefully review the written treatment plan summary. They usually gather a different set of insights from listening to the recording than those they received while in the session.

Finally, the health guide meets with the patient within two weeks of the Healing Circle. In this important meeting, the two review the Circle's overall outcome, reconsider its written recommendations, and refine the treatment plan. Periodically, additional sessions may be held, depending on the patient's needs and wishes and on the health guide's judgment.

The following story is a representative example of a Healing Circle recently held at HMC.

At a high point of enjoying her life at age 67, "Sally" discovered a lump in her left breast and came to our clinic. We performed a mammogram that indicated the likelihood of a cancer. Sally agreed to have it biopsied, which revealed a 1-centimeter invasive carcinoma. After consultation with her surgeon and two oncologists, I notified her that she might need surgery and perhaps chemotherapy and radiation, in combination with CAM therapies. Sally was, quite understandably, overwhelmed and terrified.

Over the next few weeks, she and her husband, Roger, began a frantic Internet research project and found their situation more challenging than they had anticipated. Their research also included consultations with a naturopath who had advanced experience with cancer treatments, a psychologist, and a specialist in interactive guided imagery—all members of our Health Medicine Center staff. Sally and Roger now felt better educated, but they explained to me that they were getting conflicting messages from this myriad of specialists regarding the best treatment; they felt confused, upset, and even a bit disempowered as to how to make the right decisions about treatment. They were also quite apprehensive about conventional cancer therapy. To resolve this complex situation, so typical with the difficult disease of cancer, I offered to bring her entire team of practitioners together, including her surgeon and lead oncologist, into a Healing Circle with both Sally and Roger present. Everyone agreed to participate.

Over the two-hour session, all of the practitioners had the opportunity to present their point of view to Sally and Roger. It was interesting to learn about the practical and realistic advantages, limitations, and problems of each approach in Sally's case. As her health guide, I chaired a wide-ranging discussion about how the varied styles of therapies could come together in a personalized treatment program that would meet Sally's unique needs.

By the conclusion of the session, the group had shifted from information exchange to genuine connection. We watched as Sally became filled with the sense of how fully she was supported by the entire group. The Circle arrived at the common ground needed for creating a treatment approach that would best meet Sally's physical, emotional, and spiritual needs and preferences. Based on our recommendations, she opted for a simple mastectomy followed by a five-year course of Arimidex (a conventional oncology drug that would block the effects of estrogen on any tumor that might remain in her body), but she decided to hold off on radiation treatment. Sally and Roger also chose to work on supporting her wellness with lifestyle measures that included exercise, a low-carbohydrate diet, plenty of sunshine and vitamin D supplements, immune support, and a regular detoxification program. Eight years later, Sally is still cancer free and is delighted with her outcome. She recently told me, "Without my Healing Circle and the loving support Roger and I received, I don't know how we could have found peace in the decisions we made."

Practitioner responses to Healing Circles

You may be surprised to find that no fees are paid to Circle practitioners for their participation; our firm policy is that all such services are pro bono. This may sound impractical at first, but we have discovered that the joy of giving and the profound sense of connection experienced by everyone in Circles is usually more than enough payment. We even find that some practitioners, once they've been part of a Circle, engage in them as often as twice a month. In fact, it has been rare for invited practitioners to refuse Circle participation for any reason, including lack of compensation. And many practitioners feel that their experience is a wake-up call that something very important is missing from both mainstream and CAM practice—*giving*.

I see Circles as offering their own reward. They're a reminder that the joy of giving and of graciously accepting love *is* supremely satisfying. After all, many of us have come to believe that it is *love* that heals at the deepest level.

Additional incentives for practitioners to participate include the more "practical" benefit of assisting their own patients in developing advanced treatment plans based on multiple perspectives in an integrative setting. Practitioners also further their own professional expertise through observing the rich responses from a diverse group of colleagues to a difficult case. The overall impression of both patients and practitioners has been that Healing Circles are a deeply touching as well as cost-effective method of resolving what had been irresolvable illnesses.

Finally, Healing Circles have the potential to do more than help patients and practitioners. They could also bring substantial relief to our financially overburdened system. We used to charge $500 for each Circle—a small expense when compared, for example, with the costs of many high-tech diagnostic tests. But we changed this policy because we have come to believe that they have a greater impact when services are pro bono. Circles may even avert a hospitalization that can cost more than $150,000.

Of course, formal Healing Circles are not always indicated. We have discovered many pragmatic variations on how their principles can be utilized in a genuine integrative setting.

"Linda," for example, never had a Circle, but each of her practitioners at HMC spent considerable time discussing how to best serve her. Sometimes we did this in Linda's presence, and at other times we met without her—thus illustrating one of the many advantages of working together in the same building in common offices.

Linda was gifted with the talent to be one of the world's top tennis players. Even when I knew her as a teenager, her unusual skills were obvious. I recall how the rest of the pack of ordinary tennis players marveled at her talent; we considered her a phenom. As a junior tennis player, she won the national women's 18-year-old clay championships, with victories over Tracy Austin and Pam Shriver. She also won the U.S. Open Junior Championships. However, Linda soon discovered that she did not enjoy being on the women's professional tour because of the grueling travel schedule. She chose to become a teaching professional and live a "normal" life. Yet she still loved playing tennis.

Linda had suffered from numerous minor injuries over the past 20 years, but in 2001 she was badly injured in an auto accident, suffering a fractured right arm and severe, unrelenting pain in her neck and back. Over the next couple of years, the pain spread to her entire back as well as her arms and legs. Consultations with a series of physicians led to the conclusion that Linda was suffering from fibromyalgia. Although she was treated aggressively with a variety of drugs to relieve her intractable pain, nothing worked. In fact, the drugs interfered with her ability to function because of their side effects.

I had lost track of her, but in fall 2008, our paths crossed. Once a year she returned to the Berkeley Tennis Club to play in an exhibition pro-am tennis tournament, but this time she wasn't sure she could participate. She called and asked me if I'd test her to see if she could play. Linda told me of her misfortune and of how it had so radically changed her life. We played great tennis for about 20 minutes, and her form looked just as perfect as it had been 20 years earlier. However, her pain was soon too great and she had to stop. While still at the club, I examined her neck and low back, and it was clear that she was in severe pain. I was amazed that she could play at all. We went directly to my office, where I did a diagnostic scan of her neck and back with the photonic stimulator.

Now, Linda's personality had always been confident and positive, and she was a tough competitor. Although fibromyalgia was a possible diagnosis, somehow I knew that it did not match with the Linda I had known 20 years before. To my surprise, her scan clearly diagnosed that she had a severe problem with discs in her neck and back.

After our many conversations, HMC practitioners treated Linda over the course of the next several weeks with photonic stimulation, chiropractic adjustments, imagery, and bodywork. As of this writing, about six months later, her pain has been reduced by about 75 percent. She's able to do some of her normal activities with only minor discomfort, and she is no longer on pain medications. Linda and I are looking forward to a day when we can hit a few balls once again.

Linda's story is a good example of how important it is to know *the whole person.* It is critical to listen carefully to each person's story and evaluate all aspects of who she is—body, mind, emotion, and spirit—in the context of her entire life story. One must especially question a diagnosis arrived at when the previous practitioner did not take the time to know a patient in *all domains.* The collaborative consultations we carried out at HMC were also critical in resolving Linda's symptoms.

Can mainstream and CAM practitioners work together?

I realize that Healing Circles are futuristic—probably even far ahead of the standards of collaborative practice in most integrative centers. The fact that this exciting clinical technique has evolved only in the San Francisco Bay Area is probable evidence of the uneven progress in the acceptance of the new medicine nationwide. Still, the *general* shift from a conventional practice to one that is integrative has been agonizingly slow for large portions of the public and certainly for CAM practitioners. Ironically, the shift has been too fast for the mainstream medical industry and its political supporters, whose paradigm and income are at stake. By virtue of their fundamentalist training and separatist orientation, most physicians are not open to working together in clinical settings as a collaborative force that operates from the standpoint of multiple healing perspectives.

And almost no encouragement for change is coming to them from medical schools or from government.

Given the steadfast demand for CAM or integrative approaches from the public over several decades, this seems highly maladaptive. Today's health care industry is not adjusting to undeniable market realities, even as it continues to enrich itself on disease care practices. As we will see in the final chapter, elements in the industry collude to politically delay the promotion of preventive policies, the funding of CAM research, and legislation to support integrative solutions and create universal health care insurance—all of which are favored by a majority of Americans.

But the ethical question remains. Does the spirit of the Hippocratic Oath permit a doctor to abandon further efforts to help a patient if there is no hope from the standpoint of a single discipline? For example, should mainstream oncology physicians send their cancer patients home to die just because there are no answers from within their own paradigm? Physicians in this setting usually tell their patients that there is nothing more that modern medicine can do and that it is not worth looking elsewhere for help. Of course, many alternative practitioners make this same fatal error.

I believe such attitudes no longer work with the educated lay public. Is there anyone who is seriously ill and not getting better who would turn down a healing council where many disciplines come together to consider what might be possible from the perspective of each? In my experience, although many CAM practitioners have some resistance to truly partnering with other health care modalities to create a higher synthesis, physicians have much more resistance. The result has been a fruitless turf war waged at the expense of patients dealing with difficult health care issues.

Resolving this situation takes special people—pioneers who are willing to stretch to explore new approaches that are beyond their own training. This is what we should expect from true healers.

Without the willingness of practitioners to work as a community of healers, new possibilities will never be tested and brought forward into clinical practice.

In the end, what everyone wants is "good" medicine. It doesn't make any difference whether it comes from the mainstream or CAM, or from the East or the West. We just want the best treatment for our health problems. I find it tragic that health care practitioners from different disciplines have not found more ways to work together to provide the best care possible, especially given that no discipline by itself has found an effective way to treat any of our epidemic chronic diseases. I do acknowledge that there are many understandable reasons for this resistance. Disciplines such as Chinese medicine, homeopathy, energy medicine, and western medicine each bear radically different assumptions and technical languages; some are based on traditional Newtonian science, others on quantum physics, and still others on ancient cosmologies. Yet I believe we can and *will* learn to collaborate— I've seen it happen in practice at my own integrative clinics. And in time, we *will* overcome the chronic disease epidemic. Through the firm intention for radical reform of health care, combined with the embrace of a broader and deeper model of medicine, we can get there.

Nine

The Imperative of
Radical Health Care Reform

The crushing cost of health care . . . now causes a bankruptcy in America
every 30 seconds. By the end of the year, it could cause 1.5 million
Americans to lose their homes. In the last eight years, premiums have grown
four times faster than wages. And in each of these years, one million more
Americans have lost their health insurance. It is one of the major reasons
why small businesses close their doors and corporations ship jobs overseas.
And it's one of the largest and fastest-growing parts of our budget. Given
these facts, we can no longer afford to put health care reform on hold.

—President Barack Obama

If reform fails again, we'll be on the way to a radically unequal society, in
which all but the most affluent Americans face the constant risk of financial
ruin and even premature death because they can't pay their medical bills.

—Nobel Prize–winning economist Paul Krugman

In October 2008, a group of protesters walked into the lobby of Cigna, one of the nation's largest health insurance companies. In a single stream, they moved toward the elevators that led to its executive offices. These protestors were determined to confront the Cigna executives who had denied a liver transplant for a 17-year-old named Nataline, which led to her death. At the head of the group were Hilda and Krikor Sarkisyan, Nataline's aggrieved parents, accompanied by group of activist nurses, some of whom had been present the day Nataline died. The group alleged that the company first denied the transplant and then intentionally approved it too late to save their daughter. The protestors demanded an audience with the CEO, but as one might expect, the company instead sent out a PR manager to put them off.

One of the nurses who accompanied Nataline's parents, Donna Smith of the California Nurses Association, provides a chilling account of what happened next: "During the protest we all looked up to see a group of people looking over the mezzanine railings above us. They must have been looking down at us during the whole protest. Hilda called up, 'Do you work for Cigna?' And suddenly what we saw was too horrific to be believed. One of the young men 'flipped off' Hilda and Krikor—with gestures on both hands. We all let out a collective scream of disbelief. The young man quickly retreated from his perch. It was a moment I do not think any of us will ever forget. A Cigna employee obscenely gestures parents of a dead teenager and guess what? Cigna called the police to have the protesters removed from the lobby."[1]

This story graphically illustrates the extreme levels of conflict now built into our health care system. It shows almost cinematically that health care in the United States of America is a *commercialized, symptom-centric system* that traps all of the participants in its crazy logic—both the "victims" and the alleged perpetrators. I'll bet that whoever at Cigna pulled the plug on Nataline also feels ensnared by this logic. That's why it is *not enough* to simply blame Cigna—despite the sincerity of Nataline's supporters. Cigna may stand as an example of an insurance industry gone overboard with greed, but we need to go much deeper than simply blaming the Cignas, Aetnas, and Humanas of the world for our health care problems when such corporations are simply serving their investors within the prevailing assumptions of the disease care system.

Step back and think about it.

Would it also make sense to blame "greedy" pharmaceutical and HMO executives for our health care mess? These people are acting within the law (or up to its outer margins), and their highest duty is to maximize shareholder returns. If they failed at that, their boards would just fire them and hire other executives who *could* deliver bigger profits.

Is it fruitful to blame mainstream physicians, most of whom are unwittingly caught up in the assumptions of the disease care industrial complex, beginning from their earliest days of training—and who look at alternative medicine and see little more than economic insecurity, unhelpful regulation, incomplete research, and political hassles?

Is it fair to lay the guilt for creating our horrid health care system at the feet of our legislators, who are simply doing what politicians usually do—responding to the most powerful voices among their constituencies and acting on those issues in a way that will keep them in office?

All of these parties are functioning within the confines of a system they did not create, but inherited.

Individuals or organizations here and there within the system may be more sensitive or more service oriented than others, but their behavior does not significantly alter the core problem: We need to put a graceful end to the commercialized disease care organism itself. This begins when we challenge its scientific assumptions *from the standpoint of the new integral medicine model*, while moving toward radically reforming its flawed systems of research, regulation, financing, and delivery. We say *radical* reform because the system is broken and because the lives and health of millions of families—like that depicted on this book's cover—are now at stake.

The current debate about health care reform misses much of this diagnosis. True, government-sponsored single-payer health insurance, or some equivalent—such as the so-called "public insurance option"—makes sense on its own terms, and we should all support it in principle. But even more advanced reform is needed. We have argued in this book that the structure of disease care is too often wasteful, counterproductive, inefficient, prone to corruption, and even lethal. Do we really want to pool the health care insurance premiums of the entire population so as to better finance *this* system while leaving its other assumptions unchallenged—especially if these assumptions drive up costs beyond all reason and don't deliver wellness, prevention, and healing? And by the same token, do we really want to "automate" disease care with billions of government dollars now being targeted for information technology, when the very foundations of the industry itself need reconfiguring first?

America's health care needs reform that is both *paradigmatic* and *institutional*, not just a reform of its financing mechanisms or computer tweaks in the flow of medical information. In short, we believe the nation needs radical health care reform based on the *integral-health medicine model*.

Aside from being informed by the integral worldview,[2] the new model should be dominated by a philosophy of prevention and wellness, and financed by a single-payer universal health insurance system. Integral-health medicine as a system would permit maximal freedom to choose one's therapeutic approach according to personal preferences and the sacred bond between patient and physician. It would incorporate integrative or holistic approaches at every juncture—especially for reasons of cost-effectiveness—and it should robustly fund truly objective, comparative, and broad-ranging scientific research that's not compromised by corporate influence. This futuristic approach to health care would train physicians to be humanistic, humble, compassionate, and spiritually aware. It would incorporate deep considerations about environmental, agricultural, and even social and cultural influences on health. And it would insist on thorough reform of the FDA.

And that's the short list!

The debate always continues, but we believe that such a composite of radical reforms would represent the systemic change we need and catalyze a genuine return to healing.

All the many details about such "health care change we can believe in" could fill another book, but in this chapter we will consider the debate about national insurance in the context of the overarching issues of paradigm change and institutional transformation, and in the light of the many ancillary issues discussed in this book.

But first, let's review a few fundamentals about the costs and quality of the delivery of health care services.

A last look at the health care cost catastrophe

The key reason for America's health care cost dilemma should by now be clear: Disease care usually involves fighting the wrong war, or what might be called after-the-fact warfare. We are devoting vastly more resources to treating ill health than to health promotion and prevention—at least 25 times more. Essentially, we're not focused on the true causes of our health problems.

Our lack of prevention services is dreadful: As many as half of all Americans do not even receive the most rudimentary preventive care, such as screens for diabetes, hypertension, or cancer— even blood pressure checks. A great deal of unnecessary illness and suffering results from this neglect, and worse, the trail ends with over 100,000 *preventable deaths* each year. Leaving aside the direr statistics on iatrogenic deaths cited in chapter 4, that figure still puts the United States at 19th in the category of preventable deaths worldwide—or *last place* among industrialized nations. Our deficit in preventive care and wellness orientation means that far more money must be spent on helping these neglected people *after* their untreated conditions have become acute—that is, if they don't die first.

Of the more than $2 trillion we pour into health care each year, "a frightening 75 cents of every dollar goes towards treating patients with chronic illnesses," wrote Kenneth Thorpe, chair of the Department of Health Policy at Emory University, in the *Huffington Post* in February 2009. "In Medicaid, this figure is an even more regrettable 83 cents of every dollar; in Medicare, it's an astounding 96 cents." He continued, "The outlook is grim for finding a solution to stem rising health costs short of helping Americans transform their unhealthy behaviors."[3]

It is refreshing to see the rudimentary steps that the Obama administration is taking to emphasize prevention and comparative effectiveness research (i.e., independent comparisons of the effectiveness of the leading medical treatment options for each disease), but much more is needed if we are to obtain a reasonable return on our health care investment.

The moral problem with private health insurance

Also by way of review, let's look one last time at America's health insurance numbers.

In all industrialized countries except ours, every citizen is automatically covered in some form of single-payer system. In our fragmented private-public insurance system, an unacceptable 15 percent of all Americans are entirely uninsured, and vast numbers are underinsured. As President Obama pointed out in the quote at the top of this chapter in his address to Congress on February 14, 2009, about a million Americans fall away each year from full coverage as their premiums go up, and it's no wonder: Premiums rose four times faster than wages during the years of the Bush presidency. Over the past five years, Obama also said, premiums have risen more than five times faster than the rate of inflation.

Many of these inflated costs occur at the meeting place of two implacable forces: our disease care obsession and our medical system's addiction to an expansion (in hospital and HMO settings) of new drugs, devices, tests, and procedures that might offer incremental or even no improvements to some, but which turn a high profit. A prime example: One major study of mainstream cardiology showed that angioplasties and stents do not prolong life or even prevent heart attacks in stable patients (i.e., about 95 percent of all such patients who receive them), and that bypass surgery prolongs life in less than 3 percent of patients. Yet these procedures cost $100 billion per year! Medicare and most other private insurers cover these expensive and invasive treatments, but according to an article in the *Wall Street Journal*, "they pay very little—if any money at all—for integrative medicine approaches that have been proven to reverse and prevent most chronic diseases."[4]

This illustrates, once again, that the kicker—the ultimate disgrace of disease care medicine—is our dismal and costly record of care for chronic conditions.

And even if disease care did deliver satisfactory results with the treatment of these conditions, it would be unable to distribute the results affordably. A 2008 study by the Commonwealth Fund compared adults with chronic conditions in seven major industrialized countries. A stunning 54 percent of the American respondents said they were likely to go without recommended care, finding it unaffordable, compared with just 7 percent of chronically ill patients in the Netherlands. Over 40 percent of the American patients spent more than $1,000 on medical bills on average for a given chronic condition, compared with just 4 percent of British and 5 percent of French patients.

Such data on cost-effectiveness, in addition to the accompanying scary stories of personal misfortune, lead to a sobering conclusion: To the extent that disease care, with its focus on acute care or crisis intervention, has a place in any future system—which it does in our integral-health medicine model—offering it affordably and universally is the right thing to do. America has a moral obligation to guarantee health care coverage for *all* Americans—or some sort of comprehensive health safety net. Access to care is well established worldwide as a basic right, and the majority of citizens in our country plus most physicians agree with this commonsense policy.

Of course, in our view, guaranteeing disease care coverage is a relatively small step in the right direction, when compared with the real elephant in the room.

The economic argument for universal health care

Nonetheless, let's set aside the paradigm challenge for a moment. And let's further assume that for ideological reasons, one is not swayed by the *moral* argument for universal health insurance.

Even if so, the *economic* argument for universal insurance is alone compelling.

First of all, we have shown that when one compares our health costs with those of other countries also operating largely within the disease care paradigm, national health insurance is always found to be more cost-effective and is able to deliver higher quality.

Second, we already pay dearly for the uninsured and underinsured. Those without affordable access must go *somewhere* for treatment. All over America, we find such unfortunate people clogging our emergency rooms, often for nonurgent problems, but especially when their poorly treated chronic diseases, usually a result of poor prevention practices, take a catastrophic turn. All such costs are passed on in the form of higher delivery costs for everyone.

Next, there's the onerous administrative cost of private insurance. Insurance companies spend nearly $100 billion alone just in marketing, underwriting, and billing for the varied insurance packages offered to employers, according to the McKinsey Global

Institute.[5] Compared with the costs of a single-payer system, this is pure waste and just one more example of many we have cited. No wonder the overall administrative cost of private insurance per person in the U.S. is double that of Canada.

So again, why not provide insurance for every citizen up front, thus lowering costs across the board by pooling all demand, in addition to saving money (and lives) through national programs that prevent expensive outcomes, promote healthy lifestyle, and foster integrative forms of delivery?

Perhaps the pain isn't great enough yet.

Conditions are closing in fast, though, on those who are holding out against radical health care reform. A report in *Health Affairs* estimates that if the system is left unchanged, one of every five dollars spent by Americans in 2017 will go to health care. Half of all bankruptcies in America occur because families are unable to pay their medical bills, and this number too will rise.[6] With premiums shooting up about 10 percent each year, the insurance industry is pricing itself out of the market for an ever-larger part of the population.

Apparently, the insurance giants like it that way. Can we stand up to them?

It's going to be a huge battle.

"The private health insurance companies and the pharmaceutical industry completely and totally oppose national health insurance," said Steffie Woolhandler, MD, a founder of Physicians for a National Health Program (PNHP). "The private health insurance companies would go out of business. The pharmaceutical companies are afraid that a national health program will, as in Canada, be able to negotiate lower drug prices."[7] Woolhander and many other commentators further point out that Canadians and the U.S. Department of Defense have negotiated a 40 percent reduction on the price of drugs.[8] Meanwhile, the rest of the U.S. has moved in the opposite direction: The corrupt Medicare Prescription Drug Act, passed in 2003 at the behest of Pharma lobbyists, mandated that Americans pay *retail price* for drugs that are already overpriced.

It would seem that we're facing nothing less than a titanic economic struggle between the interests of a few large industries geared to profit and the health needs of the entire American population. And the bottom-line economic issue is the very concept of private health insurance. Simply put, a single-payer system diffuses costs and risk into a vast nationwide pool; insurance provided by several hundred private companies *fragments* the risk pool, skimming off the healthier part of the population and leaving the rest uninsured or underinsured.

Scores of lobbyists for the medical-industrial-insurance complex walk the halls of Congress bewailing what might happen to their clients if we radically reform the health care system. And yet, according to a January 15, 2009, *CBS News/New York Times* poll, 59 percent of Americans surveyed said they favored single-payer insurance, almost double the 32 percent who said they were opposed. And a majority (49 percent versus 45 percent) said they would pay higher taxes to get universal coverage in a NBC News/ *Wall Street Journal* poll.

America's future solvency is threatened by the absurdly high cost of privately financed health care to the nation and the federal budget. Seasoned journalist Joe Conason put it in perspective: "In the coming decades, [European countries, as well as Canada and Japan] will be able to invest their resources in energy and education, while we try to figure out how to borrow enough to keep our hospitals open. What they all have in common is that they do not devote a huge proportion of their health spending to the profits of insurance companies—and they negotiate budgets with health providers, such as pharmaceutical companies."[9]

Universal health insurance:
a crucial debate of our time

No doubt reform of some sort is coming. But at the time of this writing, the mainstream press and the new Obama administration are virtually ignoring the single-payer option.[10] And the only intellectually serious debate today is between advocates of single-payer government-provided universal health insurance and proponents of a few market-based alternatives now in vogue in Washington. These include a voucher system called the Guaranteed Healthcare Access Plan, which allows all Americans to shop for a standardized basic package from competing private insurers, and an employer-based approach that preserves a central role for private insurance while creating a government-run pool for the uninsured that competes with private insurers (i.e., the "public option").

Let's compare these ideas with classic single-payer insurance. Senators Ted Kennedy and John Conyers—and the many cosponsors of HR 676, the United States National Health Insurance Act, which calls for universal coverage—like to call it "Medicare for all," a reminder that we already have a successful and popular single-payer program for the elderly. Single-payer plans typically involve a publicly administered fund that guarantees coverage for everyone. Private health insurers are eliminated, or their role is substantially reduced. Only government *insurance* will become public; all services, products, and delivery remain private. Patients go to the doctors and hospitals of their choice, and there are no exclusions based on ability to pay or prior conditions. As in all other developed countries, HR 676 would provide for uniform, comprehensive coverage for all citizens, including dental, vision, and long-term care.

"The great advantage of universal, government-provided health insurance is lower costs," wrote Nobel Prize–winning economist Paul Krugman in the *New York Times*. "Canada's government-run insurance system has much less bureaucracy and much lower administrative cost than our largely private system. Medicare has much lower administrative costs than private insurance does. The reason is that single-payer systems don't devote large resources to screening out high-risk clients or charging them higher fees. The savings from a single-payer system would probably exceed $200 billion a year, far more than the cost of covering all of those now uninsured." The biggest barrier to change, said Krugman, is the private insurance industry itself. "Bill Clinton's health care plan failed in large part because of a dishonest but devastating lobbying and advertising campaign financed by the health insurance industry. . . . And the lesson many people took from that defeat is that any future health care proposal must buy off the insurance lobby."[11] Nonetheless, Krugman—and a growing chorus of other economists that includes Nobel Prize winner Joseph Stiglitz—advocates that we face up to this self-interested lobby and go all the way to a single-payer system.

Physicians favor a single-payer system

Among physicians too, the tide is turning. A 2007 survey by Indiana University found that 60 percent of physicians supported government legislation to establish national health insurance—a 10 percent increase in such support since 2002.[12]

An articulate physician speaking out for change is John Geyman, MD, professor emeritus of family medicine at the University of Washington and author of *Do Not Resuscitate: Why the Health Insurance Industry is Dying, and How We Must Replace It* (Common Courage Press, 2009). "Private health insurance is obsolete," said Geyman. "Over the past 40 years, private insurance has evolved from a not-for-profit activity into a $300-billion-a-year, for-profit, investor-owned industry. The six biggest insurers made over $10 billion in profits in 2006. They did so by enrolling healthy people, denying claims, and screening out the sick, who are increasingly being shunted into our beleaguered public safety net programs. These for-profit companies have burdened our system with enormously wasteful administrative costs and skyrocketing CEO salaries, while leaving tens of millions uninsured and underinsured." Geyman continued, "The risk pool has been badly fragmented among more than 1,300 private insurers, defeating the goal of insurance, which is to provide coverage by sharing risk across a broad population."

Geyman believes the savings from a single-payer system would be far greater than the $200 billion claimed by Krugman: "The administrative savings alone would be $350 billion a year, enough to cover all of the uninsured and underinsured."[13]

In just one month in 2008, over 5,000 U.S. physicians, organized by Geyman and others, signed an open letter calling on Washington "to stand up for the health of the American people and implement a nonprofit, single-payer national health insurance system.... The incremental changes suggested by most Democrats cannot solve our problems; further pursuit of market-based strategies, as advocated by Republicans, will exacerbate them," they wrote. "What needs to be changed is the system itself."[14]

Creating health and wellness through national prevention policies

But the system may more ideologically entrenched than most of us can fathom.

For example, ask yourself: Why did President Bush in late 2007 twice veto a bipartisan bill that would have increased cigarette taxes to fund health care for ten million uninsured children?[15] Who in their right mind would decide *not* to insure our children in order to keep down the price of a product that has been proved to cause cancer, emphysema, asthma, fetal damage, heart attacks, strokes, and many other serious medical diseases, and which costs our health care system billions of dollars every year? One might pin this crazy decision on the person of the president himself, but we would submit that it reflects something far deeper—a systemic problem in America's political culture. (In a happy reversal, the new Democratic Congress and the Obama administration passed a similar bill early in 2009.)

To give a narrower example, why do we spend up to $100,000 for the care of premature babies with low birth weights when we do relatively little to address the main cause of this difficulty—smoking by pregnant women? One estimate found that a program to help pregnant women to quit would cost just $50 per woman.

Ask yourself also: Why has the federal government not taken steps to clean up the FDA and empower it to regulate pharmaceutical drugs more effectively and responsibly, even though the FDA's ability to do its job, by its own admission, has collapsed? Why has Congress protected Big Pharma from fair and proper regulation of prices and quality even though innumerable congressional investigations have shown that the FDA is riddled with conflicts of interest and incompetence?

Just follow the money, as the old saying goes.

Confident that sanity will eventually win out over corruption, we offer the following Five-Point Plan—a modest set of preventive and regulatory measures that could greatly reduce costs by making America healthier. We believe that such programs should precede or at least accompany any effort to universalize health care insurance:

1. **Fund programs that make exercise universally available and attractive.** Do we really want to reduce health care costs and improve the well-being of all Americans? Our epidemic of obesity and Type 2 diabetes has become a national emergency, and we know for a certainty that regular exercise helps prevent these maladies as well as heart disease, stroke, hypertension, fractured bones in old age, depression, and so much more. To avert such costly diseases

and maintain peak health, every child and adult should have at least *an hour a day* reserved for appropriate exercise.

- Our first priority should be to greatly upgrade the physical education and health education requirements and capabilities in all public schools; no child should be "left behind" when it comes to acquiring fitness habits that can bless him or her for a lifetime.

- As a second priority, let's make exercise more available and more attractive to every adult by providing free or inexpensive exercise facilities in every locality—in parks, recreation centers, government buildings, and businesses—and let's give incentives to citizens to use these facilities or take exercise classes in these spaces.

- Other obvious methods include incentives linked to health insurance, expansion of competitive sports, and subsidies for private-sector enterprises targeting wellness and exercise.

America can find creative and inspiring ways to motivate the population to exercise throughout life; with a relatively tiny expenditure of government funds, we can save vast amounts of money on managing diseases while also improving the physical and mental health of our people.

2. Tax junk food; subsidize sustainable agriculture, healthy foods, and supplementation. We all know that Americans are increasingly overfed and yet undernourished, and that obesity, diabetes, heart disease, cancer, and mental health problems are directly linked to diet. One way to scale back the incidence of these diseases is to *include the social and health costs* of a food in its price. We already address the cost to society of alcohol and tobacco products by adding a hefty tax to their retail price, and we ban street drugs because of their social cost and even lock up millions of people for simply using them. Why not extend this principle to the regulation of unhealthy foods and beverages that wreck the health of our children and a large percentage of adults? Here are a few methods for carrying this out:

- The first priority would be to abolish junk food in schools and hospitals, or add a "health tax" to each purchase in such locations, using these revenues to educate students and hospital patients.

- Healthier eating habits could be supported for the entire population through pervasive public education that demonstrates how eating whole foods is less expensive than consuming processed food over time. This is especially important now that the cost of fresh fruits and vegetables is climbing faster than inflation rates, making junk food relatively cheaper.[16]

- A more aggressive approach entails finding ways to provide for a *reduction* in purchase price for demonstrably healthy foods. This might be accomplished by laws or subsidies that favor organic agriculture, through trade policy, or even by offering some form of direct subsidy to consumers of health food (or perhaps food supplements).

- Toxic residues in our foods from chemical fertilizers, pesticides, and animal drugs have disastrous effects on human health, and conclusive evidence shows that factory farming has led to a decrease in the nutrient contents of fruits and vegetables. This is another strong reason for government support of organic farmers and sustainable agricultural practices, favoring them over corporate agribusiness.

- Along the same lines, let's promote or subsidize inexpensive food supplementation for the whole population. We know that nutrients such as vitamin D have indisputable disease-prevention effects. One authority called vitamin D deficiency "a national emergency" and claimed that if all Americans simply supplemented with just 1,000 IU of vitamin D$_3$ each day, this could save thousands of lives and tens of billions of dollars.[17]

Once legislative initiatives like the ones listed above got started, incentives would be in place for American industry to step up production of health-promoting products. There would be political resistance to all these ideas from industries that profit from unhealthy products, but one could also imagine support for such a program from more enlightened members of the insurance industry, fruit and vegetable producers, organizations for health promotion and prevention, the health food industry, organic farmers, and many business organizations—not to mention physicians' organizations.

3. Fund comparative assessment research of treatments and legally require disclosure of all treatments backed by scientific evidence, including CAM approaches. Another key prevention technique—one that goes beyond a related proposal in the Obama administration's health care plan at this time of writing—is legislation that mandates funding for basic research to support the comparative assessment of *all* treatments (both mainstream and CAM) that are known from evidence to be beneficial for specific diseases. This legislation would require disclosure of these findings to health care practitioners, insurers, and the public. In particular, such a law should *mandate* disclosure of all reasonable options to patients diagnosed with specific maladies. The goal of such legislation would be to support the *right to know*—a key premise of truly integrative medicine. Using such research to cut across all known mainstream and alternative techniques could be a fatal blow to the parochialism that besets the disease care model. Of course, fostering such an expansion in the nation's medical treatment repertoire is a colossal challenge, but consider these facts and issues:

- Most heart bypass surgery can be avoided by offering lifestyle programs. Such programs are widely used in Europe and have been proved effective in the United States. But very few patients in the U.S. are made aware of this option before they make decisions about cardiac interventions. Given our dire crisis in the cost of health care, why shouldn't such low-cost healthy-heart programs be widely promoted to doctors and the public, supported by insurance coverage, or in some cases possibly be mandated?[18]

- Thousands of years of experience with herbs and acupuncture in the Orient have culminated in the worldwide movement for evidence-based Chinese medicine, now typified by peer-reviewed, scientific journals such as *Chinese Medicine* and the World Health Organization's promotion of the Global Strategy for Traditional Medicine, which not only fully document the success of Oriental remedies for myriad diseases, but also recommend implementation of these healing strategies worldwide. Why aren't Americans given the option for routine access to these proven treatments, along with insurance coverage for them? *Indeed, insurance companies should be required to reimburse for health care services delivered by any health care practitioner who is licensed by the state.*

- Similarly, it is widely known that patients suffering from musculoskeletal pain respond well to massage, stretching exercises, chiropractic adjustment, and better diet—not to mention emerging technologies such as the photonic stimulator we use at the Health Medicine Center. We've discussed in this book the known risks of Big Pharma's painkillers used so widely to manage musculoskeletal and other forms of pain. The lack of access by these patients to preventive options or other proven therapeutic options leads to innumerable injuries and deaths every year from the unnecessary use of painkillers.

4. Broadly support preventive screens. Let's make preventive screens for such conditions as high blood pressure, diabetes, and cancer routinely available and inexpensive for all citizens. Doing such tests *before* clinical disease sets in can help stop silently progressing and potentially lethal health problems in their tracks. Advanced screens have the potential to uncover important occult disease, as we saw in the cases of Pete Wilson and Tim Russert in chapter 6. At the Health Medicine Center, we routinely offer breast thermography, extremity arterial testing, heart rate variability testing, oxidative stress testing, dark field microscopy, Bio-Energy Testing, and other tests as preventive measures. Why not subsidize or fully insure tests like these for all Americans or even mandate them for certain groups, to greatly lower the cost of health care and save lives? Why not get to the true causes of a disease before the horse gets out of the barn? Recall also the importance, discussed also in chapter 6, of measuring the reserve function of our organ systems—a superior approach compared with simply screening for symptoms of advanced disease.

5. Ban DTC ads for drugs; advertise healthy lifestyle. We've noted that America remains the only country besides New Zealand that allows direct-to-consumer (DTC) TV advertising of medications. This has virtually doubled the share of today's health dollar devoted to pharmaceuticals, with up to 50 percent of prescriptions now due to patient request rather than a professionally determined need.[19] We need to turn this phenomenon on its head, perhaps with TV and radio ads that encourage and support a *healthful lifestyle*. To fund this, DTC ads by pharmaceutical companies could be taxed to contribute to a fund (perhaps matched by public funds) that would deliver equally attractive *health-promotion messages* through the same media channels. Or perhaps better yet, DTC ads should be abolished outright for being intrinsically deceptive and unethical.

Again, this is a short list; so much more can be done to boost prevention. Underlying all such measures is the paradigm shift we have discussed in this book—our rediscovery that there is no need to fight Mother Nature. It is far easier, less expensive, and more productive to adapt to what nature has provided over eons to help us deal with our health challenges. "Favoring" nature, for example, entails prioritizing our body's innate self-healing capacity, as advocated by Beauchamp in the debate between him and Pasteur that we summarized in chapter 3. Remember, the best-known precursor of our epidemic of chronic diseases is chronic inflammation. Thus, pursuing detoxification and living a healthy lifestyle using natural foods and treatments remains the best approach for both preventing and treating inflammation. Public health programs that creatively present this simple message to our citizens need to be expanded.

In line with this principle, in chapter 4 we noted that the methodology of Health Medicine requires that the least invasive therapy is the place to start. We've shown in this book why this approach, so essential to the integral model of medicine, is cost-effective and can be lifesaving. This *hierarchy of treatment modalities* bears repeating, yet again.

- Lifestyle strategies such as a healthy diet, adequate sleep and exercise, stress reduction, weight control, avoidance of toxic exposures, and securing emotional and spiritual balance in life are the *first line of defense.*

- Noninvasive complementary and alternative (CAM) services such as acupuncture, herbal medicine, chiropractic, bodywork, homeopathy, and energy medicine are *the next line of defense.*

- Natural-medicine approaches based on the latest advances in orthomolecular medicine, functional medicine, and bioenergetic research—and inclusive of the more advanced forms of testing—are a *further line of defense.*

- Very careful and sparing use of pharmaceutical drugs, surgery, and other invasive strategies are *the last line of defense.*

Once again, the new medicine does not and cannot exclude today's high-tech miracles. Quite to the contrary, the integral model of medicine supports them as long as they remain in their place in the treatment hierarchy. The very concept of integral-health medicine reserves high-tech medicine as a backup for those times when wellness and prevention and less-invasive natural therapies fail.

Integrative health care and federal health policy

For the most part, the public is driving the paradigm shift to the new medicine. This is evidenced by the way it spends its dollars—almost all of them out of pocket—on preventive measures in daily life, on integrative clinics and spas, on scores of alternative and natural treatments, on organic and fresh foods, on food supplements, and on other products and services of the burgeoning wellness market. It is far past time for Washington and the health policy establishment to catch up with this huge and growing mass of pioneers who are mapping the future of health care—and who are often their most affluent and thoughtful constituents.

Fortunately, many physicians and nurses have also caught the trend. Those now in early stages of training grew up amid the grassroots shift to holistic health and integrative medicine, and they are showing strong interest in these alternatives. As evidence of this, many medical students are requesting courses in CAM, and most medical schools are now at least providing some elective CAM courses. Students at some medical schools have even formed organizations to foster the development of a medical curriculum that offers a wide range of CAM services. Among nurses, the acceptance of the American Holistic Nurses Association by the American Nurses Association as a recognized specialty society is another sign of the times.

Andrew Weil, MD, has developed a two-year postgraduate program in integrative medicine at the University of Arizona's Health Sciences Center, which has grown substantially over the past decade and is now producing physicians who are becoming leaders nationwide, including taking positions as professors at some prestigious medical schools. Weil's books and TV shows have had a major impact on the acceptance and growth of integrative medical practice, as has the work of many other integrative physicians, such as Rachel Naomi Remen, James Gordon, Richard Kunin, Dean Ornish, Mehmet Oz, Mark Hyman, Martin Rossman, Keith Block, and scores of others.

Integrative and CAM centers are becoming more common nationwide, especially in affluent areas. Most major cities in the U.S. have several integrative medical centers that are popular and even financially solvent. Some major teaching medical centers and a few private hospitals are now offering CAM services such as bodywork, guided imagery, chiropractic, acupuncture, and Chinese herbal therapies. Notable among these are Beth Israel Medical Center's new Department of Integrative Medicine, Duke Medical Center, the University of Michigan, UCSF, and California Pacific Medical Center.

This movement is becoming substantive, yet most CAM services provided by these centers are not insured. *Now is the time to modernize insurance coverage so that it extends the integrative medicine revolution to everyone.*

Over many years, I've witnessed a painfully slow but steadily growing trend in the medical insurance industry to reimburse CAM services and products; chiropractic and acupuncture are the most notable examples. Even Medicare is beginning to offer reimbursement for some CAM services. But for innumerable healing molalities and supports such as herbs, supplements, most forms of natural medicine, and many other noninvasive natural therapies such as meditation, biofeedback, bodywork, and guided imagery, the changes in insurance policy are still far behind the science and the market demand.

Much more needs to happen in this regard, and soon. And policymakers need to impress upon the insurance industry, both publicly funded and privately run, that it is tardy in accepting the science and the empirical experience that now validates much of CAM. One quick fix to get the ball rolling could be uniform standards nationwide; reimbursed CAM services now vary substantially from company to company and from state to state.

There can be no doubt about it: Reimbursement for evidence-based integrative health care services of every kind must be liberalized, and research needs to be a high priority. Toward this end, *we need to greatly accelerate federally funded research (including comparative assessment research) into CAM at the NIH's National Center for Complementary and Alternative Medicine*, whose work is still an embarrassingly small portion of the NIH's overall budget. As we noted in chapter 5, such public funding is crucial, because the private sector will only fund medical research that lends itself to patents or to profits. The NIH in this respect remains far behind the paradigm shift that has already occurred among the American population.

All across the board, the evolution of institutions that embody the new medicine is proceeding somewhat more slowly than the unfolding of the worldview shift to integrally informed health care. And this is no doubt because of the hegemonic practices of the disease care system. Further evidence for this delayed institutional evolution is the fact that the majority of integrative and CAM centers are simply locations where practitioners of different disciplines locate their offices, as we've noted. There are only a few that are truly integral—that is, that actually practice collaboratively as we do at the Health Medicine Center. But business models like ours for creating sustainable clinics that embody the best innovations of integral medicine are waiting in the wings.

In the final analysis, the institutional changes we need are delayed by politicians still fiddling with incremental changes while the state of America's health care burns to the ground. Activists, progressive politicians, and thoughtful health policy makers will have to step in and organize the popular will needed to get federal support for integrative care for *all* Americans. The long-term success of integrative methodologies will depend, at a minimum, on their efforts to expand prevention, fund publicly funded research into CAM, and institute universal insurance coverage. In time, innovations such as integrative clinics and Healing Circles will spread everywhere throughout the health care system, bringing advanced benefits to millions of Americans and reducing costs.

Radical reform of the FDA is urgently needed

A landmark article about the FDA, "Ending the Atrocities," appeared in the March 2009 issue of *Life Extension*, written by William Faloon, director of the Life Extension Foundation. LEF, a large membership organization and manufacturer of supplements, is our nation's longest-running and most courageous critic of the FDA. In this devastating piece, Faloon called for urgent and radical reform of the FDA in order to stop its "state-sponsored carnage of the American citizenry." Sounds a bit shrill, no? It does indeed, until you learn about the FDA's appalling record of fraud and abuse and its actual admission of its own incompetence, which we mentioned in early chapters. Let's consider some key elements of Faloon's indictment of the FDA.

- **Fraudulent approval of the drug Ketek.** The FDA approved Ketek to treat pneumonia, disregarding the fact that it can also cause sudden and very serious liver damage—even approving a pediatric clinical trial of the drug involving infants as young as six months. To persuade an outside scientific advisory committee to recommend full approval, the FDA knowingly allowed a fraudulent safety study to be presented, according to a Senate investigative committee. FDA employees literally presented fake data to this committee, even as a separate criminal investigation discovered that the clinic where the study occurred was *closed* during the time it supposedly took place! Soon thereafter, the person who conducted the nonexistent "study" was criminally indicted and sentenced to almost five years in jail. Yet the FDA continued to cite this data publicly long after the principal investigator admitted it was fraudulent.

- **An unethical ban of the safest form of estrogen.** In 2008, the FDA banned the safest form of estrogen, known as *estriol*. Amazingly, the FDA had no qualms about publicly stating that its ban on estriol was based on a petition filed by Wyeth, the maker of dangerous drugs that directly *compete* with estriol— Premarin and Prempro—which we examined at the close of chapter 6. Wrote Faloon: "The FDA openly seeks to protect Wyeth's market share by denying American women access to natural estriol."

- **A revolving door and a clogged approval process.** A 2008 Associated Press report cited by Faloon revealed that a record number of FDA employees have been leaving the agency to go to work for pharmaceutical companies. According to the AP, these FDA staffers have been resigning in order to go into the "more lucrative side" of the business. The FDA's brain drain and revolving-door problem are key reasons among many, said Faloon, that explain "why the FDA drug approval process has always been a bureaucratic quagmire, where life-saving medications languish for years, decades, and sometimes forever. The drug pipeline has been 'clogged' for almost 50 years." Faloon cited *Wall Street Journal* data showing that the number of new drug approvals has fallen dramatically. The FDA approved just 16 new drugs in 2007 and 24 in 2008, down from 139 in 1996. A mixed blessing, from another point of view.

- **A lethally slow response to Paxil.** The same Senate committee uncovered yet another study with falsified data that was used to support the approval of a popular antidepressant drug called Paxil in 1991. It found that the maker of Paxil improperly put people who had previously attempted suicide into the placebo group in its clinical study. This made it appear that the Paxil group would have a suicide rate that was the same as or even lower than that of the placebo recipients. But because of FDA foot dragging, it took until 2006 for the manufacturer to send a letter to doctors admitting—once the data was rectified—that the risk of suicidal behavior was actually almost *seven times higher* in study subjects taking Paxil compared with placebo.

- **The FDA wasted millions on a broken computer system to track side effects.** Postapproval surveillance of a new drug is critical to identifying side effects not detected in the clinical trials because of the short duration of most trials. Yet the FDA squandered $25 million on a failed computer system to track side effects of approved drugs. As a result, says Faloon, "the FDA will have to rely on the previous dysfunctional system to track what are record-breaking numbers of adverse reports being made about drugs the agency previously approved as safe."

In 1994, the Life Extension Foundation established the FDA Museum to document how the FDA's failings were responsible for "the needless deaths of millions of Americans." Every assertion the foundation made about the FDA back then, said Faloon, "has been validated by third parties and the FDA itself."

With the FDA's credibility at its worst ever, there has never been a better time to enact legislation to reform it from the ground up. Among the key initiatives to do so is the work of the people at Life Extension, who are partnering with the American Association for Health Freedom, a coalition of integrative physicians, health care consumers, and health freedom activists committed to a complete reform of the FDA. Its Reform FDA Petition is available for signing at ReformFDA.org.

Making medical freedom a constitutional right

A closely related issue that must be tackled, hopefully long before we get to single-payer universal health care, is the patients' *right to freedom of choice*. We've already broached this issue just above under the rubric of *the right to know*, and also in chapter 7 in terms of patient-centered care—one of the core principles of Health Medicine. It's well worth stating again: Whom are we kidding when, because of monopolistic practices, patients are not informed of all the treatments known from evidence to benefit their condition? What's the point of extending insurance to all Americans if they're blocked from making choices outside the disease care paradigm—indeed, services and products that much of the population now demands and believes in?

America is "the land of the free," yet the public is largely unaware of the state of affairs relating to medical freedom issues. Most people are shocked when they learn that it is a felony in California for a medical doctor to prescribe a nutritional therapy as a treatment for cancer. Technically, it is even a felony for a physician to treat a patient for cancer using prayer. The only legal therapies permitted for treatment of cancer in California are surgery, radiation, and chemotherapy. This flies in the face of all logic and voluminous scientific literature.

Some therapies must, by law, be administered against people's will, despite personal or religious beliefs that may be different from mainstream thinking. Health authorities can and do take children from their parents when certain therapies are refused. They can be placed into the custody of the state, put in foster homes, and forcibly administered those therapies deemed to be essential for life.

The case of HIV-positive children is a clear example of this. If as a parent you refuse to administer the drug AZT to your child, child protective services has the right to take your child from you, put him or her in a foster home, and then forcibly administer the drug. And it's not as though the treatment is harmless. Some children die from it; AZT is a poison as well as a treatment. Even though the rationale for using this therapy is controversial, treatment of these children is still mandatory because AZT is the accepted mainstream treatment for this condition.

Similar tactics occur with certain types of cancer when they afflict children. Not only is treatment with chemotherapy mandated by law in these cases, but also alternative therapies are forbidden. A case in point is medulloblastoma, a cancer of the brain that is poorly responsive to surgery, radiation, and chemotherapy. These unfortunate children almost uniformly die within a few months to a couple of years with or without treatment. Parents who do their homework often conclude that there are sound alternatives, or that conventional chemotherapies are ineffective, toxic, and likely to traumatize their children in their final months of life. Yet, parents usually have no option except to go along with this therapy or face having their child removed and the treatment forcibly administered.

What makes this more tragic is that a well-evidenced alternative exists. A doctor named Stanislaw Burzynski long ago discovered and documented a nontoxic, safe, and often effective treatment for children with medulloblastomas, as detailed in a chapter called "The Fiercest Battle" in Daniel Haley's book *Politics in Healing*.[20] One brave family, we learn, filed a lawsuit against the physicians who failed to inform them about Burzynski's alternative treatment of brain cancer for their daughter. After these physicians performed surgery and administered radiation therapy, the family heard about the Burzynski Research Institute and its success in treating this type of brain tumor. They decided to take the child to Burzynski's clinic in Texas, and the cancer was then successfully treated. Unfortunately, however, it is reported that the child later died from the effects of the radiation previously given by her mainstream doctors.

The original physicians apparently knew about Burzynski's clinic but failed to inform the family of this option.

Now, all of us would agree that our medical authorities are well-intentioned individuals who are motivated to help us, not to hurt us. But what if, after you had researched an alternative therapy intensively, you preferred to use this therapy instead of what is required by law? You and your child or loved one would be out of luck. That's why freedom of choice is high on the agenda of radical health care reform and should even rise to the level of a constitutional right. As we have argued, genuine freedom in these matters calls for greatly expanded research into CAM, including comparative assessment, full disclosure to patients of all treatments supported by science, and insurance coverage for all such remedies—and not just for treatments supported within a disease care paradigm marred by conflicts of interest and questionable science.

Revisiting freedom of choice and "evidence-based" medicine

The story of the Burzynski clinic highlights another reason why medical freedom is essential: the mainstream paradigm's bogus claims to "solid science," which we examined in chapter 3.

Let's think about this logically. If these treatments are so solid, why do these so-called evidenced-based therapies often change drastically? For example, how many ballyhooed drugs have come and gone, often withdrawn because they didn't work or produced severe side effects? How many surgical procedures are no longer used for whatever reason? How many procedures, as we saw in the case of the earlier-cited studies of cardiology, simply don't work? How many other vaunted remedies worked because of their placebo effect, which later wore off? If all this advanced research is correct in the first analysis, shouldn't it be correct always? And if modern medicine is so advanced and "scientific," why do we have so many uncontrolled chronic diseases, not to mention hundreds of thousands of iatrogenic deaths each year?

A prime example of the need for humility is the way that mainstream medicine has managed breast cancer. The Halsted radical mastectomy is a classic example. This is a mutilating surgery that was practiced in mainstream medicine for nearly three-quarters of a century as the gold standard for breast cancer treatment. Eventually, studies proved that it offers no survival advantage over simple removal of just the breast cancer lump itself—a lumpectomy. Tragically, this surgery is still used on rare occasions.

Today, the Halsted radical mastectomy is considered bad medicine. Yet tens of thousands of women were unnecessarily subjected to it, all under the assumption that "this is the best therapy for breast cancer."

What much of evidence-based medicine turns out to mean is that treatments are based upon what we *think* we know and what we *hope* may not be counterproductive or injurious, within the confines of today's reductionist, disease care paradigm. It is more ethical to acknowledge that some guesswork is involved in medicine. It is more honest to bear in mind that knowledge evolves and current science is never "final." It is indeed a great irony that mainstream medicine holds health care disciplines that are outside its domain to overinflated standards of scientific research that it erroneously assumes are being used in its own research. In the future, when the integral model is better understood and applied, and when health care regulation is more enlightened, medical science will be based upon a pluralistic method. Such a method will consider all possibilities from all healing systems, test them impartially with an eye to their safety and cost-effectiveness, systematically inform the public of research results, cover the best-evidenced treatments with universal insurance, and permit patients the right to choose from among many reasonable options in an imperfect world.

The ultimate front line of health care: profit versus service

The old and dying paradigm of disease care medicine is deeply rooted in our culture, which currently elevates the profit motive over the simple desire to serve—even over scientific truth and professional integrity. It will probably remain so until we become oriented to honoring service before material gain and truth over self-aggrandizement. We will always face economic issues in health care; but if we find the inspiration to work together, with our highest goal being to provide service, reform will evolve naturally and appropriately.

Health care has become an enormous business, and the proper goal of businesses is to sell products and services to make money for shareholders. Private industry and commerce have a real place in health care, and properly regulated markets are a blessing to humankind. But "free markets" don't work when it comes to providing public utilities like roads and fire departments. They are far less efficient when it comes to disseminating public goods such as preventive education for healthy lifestyle, health insurance, medical choice, and the best-evidenced health care treatments. We have demonstrated in this book that overly commercialized medical care, privatized health insurance, and the untrammeled worship of free markets—combined with a materialist and reductionist model of human health that leads to a war on nature—are directly responsible for causing America to slide nearly to last place worldwide among advanced nations in the overall quality of its health care. And it is literally bankrupting the American government.

We simply cannot allow this tragic state of affairs to continue.

It is therefore time for us to take clear and powerful action. It is time to come together as peaceful warriors whose mission is to rescue the soul of medicine, fighting for what we believe in, struggling in noble service to others—even our opponents. We can fight with our votes to transform the legislation that regulates our health care industry. With our determination to find a solution to skyrocketing health care costs. With our compassion to find a better way to practice medicine. With our willingness to take back responsibility for living a healthy lifestyle. And with our commitment to bringing the *care* back into health care.

Who will step forward with the solution for our dilemma? Many open-minded healer-physicians are courageously riding the crest of a tidal wave that is sweeping across America, exposing its narcissistic, profit-driven disease care system for what it is. Their willingness to return to healing leads these caring physicians and practitioners to serve with a whole heart. It even opens a sacred space of authentic meeting with their patients and colleagues. All across this land, genuine healers are joining in partnership with humanitarians and activists who have made it their purpose in life to radically reform the institutions of health care and build a sustainable civilization. Together these leaders boldly acknowledge the importance of treating body, mind, and spirit—the imperative of caring for the whole person, not just the disease. They are choosing prevention, wellness, natural solutions, and the integrative model—and they are blazing the path to the integral-health medicine of the future.

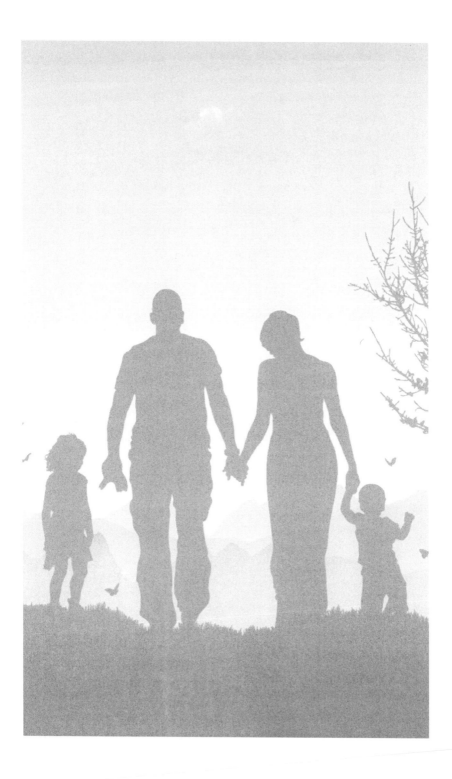

Epilogue: The Spirit of Healing

Not long ago, I was honored to participate in a *Yuwipi* ritual, an extraordinary Lakota/Sioux healing ceremony. This demanding ceremony is very hard on the healer-shamans who specialize in conducting them; these noble souls willingly sacrifice a piece of their own life force every time it is performed. It is said that Yuwipi healers lead short, difficult lives that are consecrated to the healing needs of their communities.

This particular ceremony was conducted over a period of three days on behalf of two sick infants. One of the infants had *congenital pyloric stenosis*, a condition usually treated with surgery to widen the narrowed juncture between the stomach and the duodenum. The other infant had been born with a condition called *neutropenia*, a genetic disorder of the bone marrow characterized by a lack of production of white blood cells. This rare condition has no easy Western treatment.

The ceremony began as we entered a purification lodge. I had attended *sweats* before, but none anywhere near this scorching. I fell into a panic. With a rising sense of terror, I hovered low to the ground in the thick darkness to avoid the boiling heat. My ears, nose, and face felt as though they would burst into flames any second.

And the sweat had only just begun!

As I prepared to bolt for the door, the memory of why I was there suddenly flashed through my mind. The physical discomfort immediately vanished! I dropped inward, where my only thought was to pray for the children. Two hours of darkness, timelessness, and full absorption passed.

When the doors of the lodge burst open, the trance was instantly broken. Once again, I felt that ruthless sensation of searing heat. We exited, now purified for the ceremony.

From the sweat we were led to a room in whose center was an altar laden with sacred objects and flowers. In front of it was an elder shaman who had traveled from South Dakota. He was crouching on his knees, praying at the altar. I noticed that his wrists were tied behind his back, with each finger wrapped individually in rawhide and then bound to the other fingers in such a way that all were connected. Next to him was an assistant holding a sacred pipe. Seated all around him were drummers, chanters, and people with rattles—about 20 Native Americans in all.

The lights were turned off and the pitch-black room felt eerie. Now, following the shaman's cues, the drummers drummed and the chanters chanted in unison, all against the backdrop of the rattles. As the energy in the room rose, static electricity burst in sparks from the rattles all around the darkened room. I once again became mesmerized, falling into a trance. At some point, a strange feeling entered me—somehow I *knew* that the spirits of these people had appeared in order to heal the children. As the ceremony came to an end, the lights exploded back on. We could all see that the shaman was freed of his bonds. He turned to us and stated that the spirits had freed him and that *they* had played the rattles.

This same protocol was followed for three successive nights.

Within a few weeks, we learned that the children had fully recovered without any other treatment. This was confirmed by two physicians.

If only all Americans could participate in some type of ritual or ceremony that celebrates our common humanity, so as to heal ourselves and our broken health care system!

In the world's many wisdom traditions—as in the Yuwipi ceremony—the role of spirit (and of the spirits of the celestial realms) has been revered as a vital and sacred element of the healing process. For thousands of years, spiritual guides and shamans in all cultures have passed down their mysterious healing secrets from generation to generation, and they still do. Humanity has depended on such spiritual help for millennia and continues to rely on prayer, worship, and meditation for healing—usually guided by rituals, symbols, and scriptures. The medical profession may have forgotten the central role of these spiritual aids that are nonetheless found in all known cultures—but humanity has not, and it never will.

Though mainstream medicine has not yet formally endorsed prayer or spirituality, abundant research in peer-reviewed journals documents that people with strong faith, religious belief, or consistent spiritual practices enjoy better physical, mental, and emotional health and in fact grow in their ability to self-heal. A growing subset of physicians are incorporating prayer into their armamentarium of tools, both to support themselves and to speed their patients' return to wellness.

While *spirit* can be defined in many ways, I believe it refers to an omnipresent, loving consciousness to which we—and everything in the cosmos—are inseparably connected. Our soul is the human counterpart of this same universal spirit that indwells each one of us, guiding us forward and linking us back to this universal consciousness.

As we discussed in chapter 6, healing is often referred to as a return to universal wholeness. We are indeed *single* and whole human beings, and at the same time we are integral parts, fractals, of an infinite whole that we cannot fully comprehend. Any given part of our inner life or our exterior bodily existence can be analyzed separately from all other parts, but we remain one unified entity; our body is composed of trillions of cells that operate as one, and we also have an active *interior* life in which we progress toward the oneness of cosmic consciousness, evolving through more and more advanced stages of adult maturity.

Understanding all of these dimensions is crucial in the return to healing; health practitioners of the future will view the patient through each of these windows, thereby providing more options for prevention, curing, and integral treatment. As we revise and update the meaning of holism in terms of the new findings of integral theory, integral-health medicine practitioners will look beyond physical ailments and psychological challenges to address the root causes of illness by exploring its meaning in the context of each patient's whole life story and how it relates to her family, her society, her culture, her environment, and the greater universe.

In today's more limited Western culture, we deify the mind, placing it on a pinnacle as if it alone were worthy of worship. We must overcome this obsession if we are to return to spiritual balance, peak health, and a health care system that works. Opening the heart so that we can return to our spiritual home is not a particularly mental process. The healing experience of pure consciousness—our ultimate source and center—best occurs in a state of silence, as we serenely witness the passing of thoughts and feelings, immersed in unutterable, nondual oneness with the moment. Our greatest challenge as human beings is to move beyond our narrow minds and limited culture, dipping inwardly to discern our unique, transcendent voice, which will lead us forward in our return to healing. In doing so, we will become a sacred vessel that holds all the grace and wisdom that we have the capacity to receive. It was Lao Tzu who once wrote:

> Empty yourself of everything. Let the mind become still. The ten thousand things rise and fall while the Self watches their return. They grow and flourish and then return to the source. Returning to the source is stillness, which is the way of nature.

Endnotes

Chapter 1

1. See Elisa Act, http://www.elisaact.com.
2. Trent W. Nichols and Nancy Faass, eds., *Optimal Digestive Health*, rev. ed. (Healing Arts Press), 57–65.
3. See Orthomolecular Health Medicine, http://www.ohmsociety.com.

Chapter 2

1. "Bullying Is Rife at U.S. Medical Schools," *British Medical Journal* 333 (September 30, 2006): 7570.
2. Pauline W. Chen, "Medical Student Burnout and the Challenge to Patient Care" (October 30, 2008), *New York Times.*
3. Cheryl Ulmer, Dianne Miller Wolman, Michael M. E. Johns, eds., *Resident Duty Hours: Enhancing Sleep, Supervision, and Safety* (National Academies Press/Institute of Medicine, 2008), 169.
4. Christine C. Mitchell et al., "Predicting Future Staffing Needs at Teaching Hospitals: Use of an Analytical Program with Multiple Variables," *Archives of Surgery* 142 (2007): 329–34.
5. See the Union of American Physicians and Dentists, http://www.uapd.com.

Chapter 3

1. Fortunately, a few years later, in 2004, Governor Arnold Schwarzenegger signed into law AB 1691, which protects the right of physicians to practice safe and effective alternative medicine. Acknowledging that the Medical Board of California lacked the expertise to judge the competence of CAM practitioners, this law made it legal to practice outside the mainstream, as long as patients are fully informed that the treatment being offered differs from mainstream treatments, that the treating physician does not try to persuade the patient to choose a CAM therapy over the mainstream options, and that the patient suffers no disability. This law further requires the Medical Board to create a panel of qualified CAM physicians to judge CAM services when malpractice is suspected.

2. Hannah B. Sahud et al., "Marketing Fast Food: Impact of Fast Food Restaurants in Children's Hospitals," *Pediatrics* 118, no. 6 (December 2006): 2290–97 (doi:10.1542/peds.2006-1228).

3. Leo Marcoff and Paul D. Thompson, "The Role of Coenzyme Q10 in Statin-Associated Myopathy," *Journal of the American College of Cardiology* 49, no. 23 (June 12, 2007): 2231–37.

4. We have seen how often a narrow worldview, as well as bad business practices and even corrupt politics, can override good medical science and lifesaving clinical practices. In fact, even our access to medical research has been dominated by business values that probably arise from the unhealthy politics of today's medicine. Until very recently, state- and federally funded medical research was not available without paying a sometimes expensive fee to the journals that publish this information. It wasn't until December 2008 that a bipartisan bill was passed that provides free access to everyone for National Institutes of Health (NIH) findings based on its $29 billion of funded research. Even then, the research does not have to be made public until 12 months after publication in a medical journal. It is shameful that scientific information that could lead to new strategies to help the sick is not available to everyone immediately after it is finalized by the NIH, especially when the American public itself has paid for the research studies.

5. Susie Madrak, "FDA Scientists Complain to Obama of 'Corruption,'" January 8, 2009, Truthout, www.truthout.org/010909A.

6. Office of Technology Assessment, Congress of the United States, Publication NTIS/PB-286929 (1978): 7.

7. Richard Smith, "Where Is the Wisdom? The Poverty of Medical Evidence," *British Medical Journal* 303 (1991): 798–99.

8. David A. Grimes, "Technology Follies: The Uncritical Acceptance of Medical Innovations," *Journal of the American Medical Association* 269 (1993): 3030–33.

9. Lenard I. Lesser et al., "Relationship between Funding Source and Conclusion among Nutrition-Related Scientific Articles," *PLoS Medicine* (January 9, 2007).

10. Harlan M. Krumholz et al., "What Have We Learnt from Vioxx?" *British Medical Journal* 334 (January 20, 2007): 120–23 (doi:10.1136/bmj.39024.487720.68), http://www.bmj.com/cgi/content/full/334/7585/120.

11. Marcia Angell, "Drug Companies and Doctors: A Story of Corruption," *New York Review of Books* 56, no. 1 (January 15, 2009).

12. Joan M. Lappe et al., "Vitamin D and Calcium Supplementation Reduces Cancer Risk: Results of a Randomized Trial," *American Journal of Clinical Nutrition* 85, no. 6 (June 2007): 1586–91.

13. Ushma S. Neill, "Stop Misbehaving!" *Journal of Clinical Investigation* 116, no. 7 (2006): 1740–1.

14. Angell, "Drug Companies and Doctors."

15. Eric G. Campbell, et al., "Institutional Academic–Industry Relationships," *JAMA* 298 (2007): 1779–86.

16. William Faloon, "The FDA Indicts Itself," *Life Extension* (July 2008), www.lef.org.

17. For comprehensive information on the NHANES, see http://www.cdc.gov/nchs/products/elec_prods/subject/nhanes1.htm.

18. For more information on *The Nationwide Food Consumption Survey 1977–78*, see http://www.ars.usda.gov/SP2UserFiles/Place/12355000/pdf/77nfcs.pdf.

19. Pablo Monsivais and Adam Drewnowski, "The Rising Cost of Low-Energy-Density Foods," *Journal of the American Dietetic Association* 107, issue 12 (December 2007): 2071–76.

20. Randall Fitzgerald, *The Hundred-Year Lie: How to Protect Yourself from the Chemicals That Are Destroying Your Health* (New York: Dutton, 2006), 36.

21. Environmental Working Group, "Body Burden," http://www.ewg.org/reports/bodyburden1/.

22. Angell, "Drug Companies and Doctors."

23. Fitzgerald, *The Hundred-Year Lie*, 39.

24. Oliver A. H. Jones, Mahon L. Maguire, and Julian L. Griffin, "Environmental Pollution and Diabetes: A Neglected Relationship," *Lancet* 371, issue 9609 (January 26, 2008): 287–88, http://www.thelancet.com/journals/lancet/article/PIIS0140-6736(08)60147-6/fulltext.

25. Iain A. Lang et al., "Association of Urinary Bisphenol A Concentration with Medical Disorders and Laboratory Abnormalities in Adults," *JAMA* 300, no. 11 (September 17, 2008): 1303–10.

26. Niall Dickson and Jennifer Dixon, "Making the NHS Cost Effective," *Lancet* 367, issue 9525 (June 3, 2006): 1802–3.

27. Quoc V. Nguyen, "Hospital-Acquired Infections," *eMedicine*, http://emedicine.medscape.com/article/967022-overview.

Chapter 4

1. WHO, "World Health Organization Assesses the World's Health Systems" (June 21, 2000), *http://www.who.int/whr/2000/media_centre/press_release/en/print.html.

2. "The French Lesson in Health Care," *BusinessWeek* (July 9, 2007).

3. Arnold Relman, *A Second Opinion: Rescuing America's Health Care* (Public Affairs, 2007), 18.

4. Donald L. Barlett and James B. Steele, *Critical Condition: How Health Care in America Became Big Business—and Bad Medicine* (Doubleday, 2004).

5. See http://www.obesityinamerica.org/statistics/index.cfm.

6. Jason Lazarou, Bruce H. Pomeranz, and Paul N. Corey, "Incidence of Adverse Drug Reactions in Hospitalized Patients: A Meta-analysis of Prospective Studies," *JAMA* 279 (April 15, 1998): 1200–5.

7. Lucian L. Leape, "Error in Medicine," *JAMA* 272, no. 23 (December 21, 1994): 1851–57.

8. Gary Null et al., "Death by Medicine," *LifeExtension*, http://www. lef.org.

9. *Cost and Quality of Health Care: Unnecessary Surgery* (Government Printing Office, 1976). Cited in G. B. McClelland, Foundation for Chiropractic Education and Research, "Testimony to the Department of Veterans Affairs' Chiropractic Advisory Committee" (March 25, 2003).

10. A. L. Siu et al., "Inappropriate Use of Hospitals in a Randomized Trial of Health Insurance Plans," *New England Journal of Medicine* 315, no. 20 (November 13, 1986): 1259–66.

11. A. L. Siu, W. G. Manning, B. Benjamin, "Patient, Provider and Hospital Characteristics Associated with Inappropriate Hospitalization," *American Journal of Public Health* 80, no. 10 (October 1990): 1253–56.

12. B. O. Eriksen et al., "The Cost of Inappropriate Admissions: A Study of Health Benefits and Resource Utilization in a Department of Internal Medicine," *Journal of Internal Medicine* 246, no. 4 (October 1999): 379–87.

13. See Science-Based Medicine, http://www.sciencebasedmedicine. org/?p=136.

14. Eduardo Porter, "Japanese Cars, American Retirees," *New York Times*, May 19, 2006.

15. James E. Dalen, "Health Care in America: The Good, the Bad, and the Ugly," *Archives of Internal Medicine* 160 (September 2000): 2573–76.

16. Tom Daschle, Scott S. Greenberger, and Jeanne M. Lambrew, *Critical: What We Can Do About the Health-Care Crisis* (Thomas Dunne Books, 2008), 12.

17. The Kaiser Family Foundation, *National Survey of Physicians Part I: Doctors on Disparities in Medical Care* (2002), http://www.kff. org/minorityhealth/loader.cfm?url=/commonspot/security/get-file.cfm&PageID=13955.

18. Erica Frank et al., for the Society of General Internal Medicine Career Satisfaction Study Group, "Career Satisfaction of U.S. Women Physicians: Results from the Women Physicians' Health Study," *Archives of Internal Medicine* 159 (1999): 1417–26.

19. Commonwealth Fund, *Kaiser/Commonwealth 1997 National Survey of Health Insurance*, Survey Months: November 1996– March 1997, http://www.commonwealthfund.org/surveys.

20. Commonwealth Fund, "New Survey Finds Rising Numbers of Uninsured in Moderate- and Middle-Income American Families" (April 26, 2006).

21. WebMD, "CEO Compensation: Who Said Health Care Is in a Financial Crisis?" (August 23, 2007), http://www.webmd.com.

Chapter 5

1. Greg Critser, *Generation Rx: How Prescription Drugs Are Altering American Lives, Minds, and Bodies* (Houghton Mifflin, 2005), 2.

2. Erica D. Brownfield et al., "Direct-to-Consumer Drug Advertisements on Network Television: An Exploration of Quantity, Frequency, and Placement," *Journal of Health Communication* 9, no. 6 (2004): 491–97.

3. Richard L. Kravitz et al., "Influence of Patients' Requests for Direct-to-Consumer Advertised Antidepressants: A Randomized Controlled Trial," *JAMA* 293, no. 16 (April 27, 2005): 1995–2002.

4. DTC Perspectives, "10 Year DTC Review Study" (August 31, 2007), http://dtcperspectives.com/blog/?m=200708.

5. Rita Rubin, "How Did Vioxx Debacle Happen?" *USA Today* (October 12, 2004).

6. Rubin, "How Did Vioxx Debacle Happen?"

7. Press releases pertaining to actions about Rezulin (troglitazone), *Diabetes Monitor*, http://www.diabetesmonitor.com/rezulin.htm.

8. Bruce M. Psaty and Curt D. Furberg, "The Record on Rosiglitazone and the Risk of Myocardial Infarction," *NEJM* 357, no. 1 (July 5, 2007): 67–69.

9. Stephanie Saul and Gardiner Harris, "Years Ago, Agency Was Warned of a Drug's Risks," *New York Times* (May 24, 2007). Also see Committee Staff Report to the Chairman and Ranking Member, Committee on Finance of the United States Senate, "The Intimidation of Dr. John Buse and the Diabetes Drug Avandia," (November 2007), http://finance.senate.gov/press/ Bpress/2007press/prb111507a.pdf.

10. Marcia Angell, *The Truth About the Drug Companies: How They Deceive Us and What to Do About It* (Random House, 2004), 11.

11. Ishani Ganguli, "Is Your Doctor in Denial?" *Washington Post* (August 28, 2007).

12. Ganguli, "Is Your Doctor in Denial?"

13. Marcia Angell, "Drug Companies & Doctors: A Story of Corruption," *New York Review of Books* 56, no. 1 (January 15, 2009).

14. Yu-Xiao Yang et al., "Long-term Proton Pump Inhibitor Therapy and Risk of Hip Fracture," *JAMA* 296, no. 24 (December 27, 2006): 2947–53 (doi:10.1001/jama.296.24.2947).

15. Gary Taubes, *Good Calories, Bad Calories: Fats, Carbs, and the Controversial Science of Diet and Health* (Anchor Books, 2007).

16. Anthony Rodgers, "Editorial: A Cure for Cardiovascular Disease? Combination Treatment Has Enormous Potential, Especially in Developing Countries," *British Medical Journal* 326 (June 28, 2003): 1407–8 (doi:10.1136/bmj.326.7404.1407).

17. For more on the Bayh-Dole Act, see http://www.cptech.org/ip/ health/bd/.

18. For more on the Hatch-Waxman Act, see http://www.cptech.org/ ip/health/generic/hw.html.

19. For more on the Prescription Drug User Fee Act, see http://www. fda.gov/cber/pdufa.htm.

20. Alison Bass, *Side Effects: A Prosecutor, a Whistleblower, and a Bestselling Antidepressant on Trial* (Algonquin Books of Chapel Hill, 2008).

21. Melody Petersen, *Our Daily Meds: How the Pharmaceutical Companies Transformed Themselves into Slick Marketing Machines and Hooked the Nation on Prescription Drugs* (Picador, 2009).

22. Marc-André Gagnon and Joel Lexchin, "The Cost of Pushing Pills: A New Estimate of Pharmaceutical Promotion Expenditures in the United States," *PLoS Medicine*, Public Library of Science (January 2008), http://medicine.plosjournals.org.

23. Angell, "Drug Companies & Doctors."

24. Jeffrey R. Lisse et al., ADVANTAGE Study Group, "Gastrointestinal Tolerability and Effectiveness of Rofecoxib versus Naproxen in the Treatment of Osteoarthritis: A Randomized, Controlled Trial," *Annals of Internal Medicine* 139, issue 7 (October 7, 2003): 539–46 [PMID: 14530224].

25. Alex Berenson and Andrew Pollack, "Doctors Reap Millions for Anemia Drugs," *New York Times* (May 9, 2007). In fact, the FDA was considering adding a black box warning due to the fact that several recent studies had shown that these drugs might actually shorten survival when used in high doses because they can contribute to causing hypertension and blood clots. See M. Henke et al., "Erythropoietin to Treat Head and Neck Cancer Patients with Anemia Undergoing Radiotherapy: Randomized, Double-Blind, Placebo-Controlled Trial," *Lancet* 362 (October 18, 2003): 1255–60; also see eMedTV, "Epoetin Alfa: What Should I Tell My Healthcare Provider?" http://aids.emedtv.com/epoetin-alfa/precautions-and-warnings-with-epoetin-alfa.html.

26. Eric G. Campbell et al., "Institutional Academic–Industry Relationships," *JAMA* 298, no. 15 (October 17, 2007): 1779–86.

27. Angell, "Drug Companies & Doctors."

28. Gardiner Harris and Benedict Carey, "Researchers Fail to Reveal Full Drug Pay," *New York Times* (June 8, 2008).

29. Ralph Moss, "Patents Over Patients," *New York Times* (April 1, 2007).

30. Daniel Haley, *Politics in Healing: The Suppression and Manipulation of American Medicine* (Potomac Valley Press, 2000).

31. Susan Kelleher and Duff Wilson, "Suddenly Sick," *Seattle Times* (June 26–30, 2005).

32. For more on *The Antihypertensive and Lipid-Lowering Treatment to Prevent Heart Attack Trial*, see http://allhat.sph.uth.tmc.edu/Forms/protocol.pdf.

33. Andrew S. Neviaser et al., "Low-Energy Femoral Shaft Fractures Associated with Alendronate Use," *Journal of Orthopaedic Trauma* 22, no. 5 (May/June 2008): 346–50.

34. Aristotle Bamias et al., "Osteonecrosis of the Jaw in Cancer after Treatment with Bisphosphonates: Incidence and Risk Factors," *Journal of Clinical Oncology* 23, no. 34 (December 1, 2005): 8580–87.

35. B. G. Durie, M. Katz, and J. Crowley, "Osteonecrosis of the Jaw and Bisphosphonates," *NEJM* 353, no. 1 (July 7, 2005): 99–102.

36. See *osteoporosis* in Wikipedia: http://en.wikipedia.org/wiki/osteoporosis.

Chapter 6

1. Paul Zane Pilzer, *The Wellness Revolution: How to Make a Fortune in the Next Trillion Dollar Industry* (Wiley, 2002).

2. David M. Eisenberg et al., "Unconventional Medicine in the United States—Prevalence, Costs, and Patterns," *NEJM* 328, no. 4 (January 28, 1993): 246–52.

3. Eisenberg et al., "Trends in Alternative Medicine Use in the United States, 1990–1997: Results of a Follow-Up National Survey," *JAMA* 280, no. 18 (November 11, 1998): 1569–75.

4. For more on the National Center for Complementary and Alternative Medicine at the National Institutes of Health, see http://www.aapa.org/manual/21-Comp-AltMed.pdf.

5. Benedict Carey, "When Trust in Doctors Erodes, Other Treatments Fill the Void," *New York Times* (February 3, 2006).

6. For more on the Health Medicine Center, see www.healthmedicinecenter.net.

7. John P. Pierce et al., "Greater Survival after Breast Cancer in Physically Active Women with High Vegetable-Fruit Intake Regardless of Obesity," *Journal of Clinical Oncology* 25, no. 17 (June 10, 2007): 2345–51.

8. Rachel Ballard-Barbash and Anne McTiernan, "Is the Whole Larger Than the Sum of the Parts? The Promise of Combining

Physical Activity and Diet to Improve Cancer Outcomes," *Journal of Clinical Oncology* 25, no. 17 (June 10, 2007): 2335–37.

9. David Spiegel et al., "Effect of Psychosocial Treatment on Survival of Patients with Metastatic Breast Cancer," *Lancet* 2, no. 8668 (October 14, 1989): 888–91.

Chapter 7

1. John Travis was the pioneering physician who first brought the term *wellness* into public awareness. See the Wellspring (http://www.thewellspring.com/).

2. See John Weeks, "NCCAM Research Spending 2005–2007 by Modality: What Are the Big 3? Any Surprises?" (October 19, 2008) at the Integrator Blog (www. theintegratorblog.com).

3. The Forum functions as a 501(c)(3) nonprofit educational foundation. Our very active board of directors meets every other week to organize its meetings, business matters, and special events. Everyone is a volunteer and no one is paid. For more information about the HMF, visit our website: www.healthmedicineforum.org.

4. Marilyn Schlitz, Tina Amorok, and Marc S. Micozzi, *Consciousness and Healing: Integral Approaches to Mind-Body Medicine* (Churchill Livingstone, 2004).

5. Candace B. Pert, *Molecules of Emotion: The Science Behind Mind-Body Medicine* (Simon and Schuster, 1999), and Martin L. Rossman, *Fighting Cancer from Within: How to Use the Power of Your Mind for Healing* (Holt Paperbacks, 2003).

6. John Robbins, *Reclaiming Our Health: Exploding the Medical Myth and Embracing the Sources of True Healing* (H. J. Kramer, 1998).

7. Rachel Sherman and John Hickner, "Academic Physicians Use Placebos in Clinical Practice and Believe in the Mind–Body Connection," *Journal of General Internal Medicine* 23, no. 1 (January 2008): 7–10.

8. Lolette Kuby, *Faith and the Placebo Effect: An Argument for Self-Healing* (Origin Press, 2001), 34.

9. J. Brent Richards, et al., "Effect of Selective Serotonin Reuptake Inhibitors on the Risk of Fracture," *Archives of Internal Medicine* 167, no. 2 (January 22, 2007): 188–94.

10. Mayo Clinic, "Antidepressants for Children: Explore the Pros and Cons" (November 15, 2008), http://www.mayoclinic.com/print/antidepressants/MH00059/METHOD=print.

11. James A. Blumenthal et al., "Effects of Exercise Training on Older Patients with Major Depression," *Archives of Internal Medicine* 159, no. 19 (October 25, 1999): 2349–56.

12. Blumenthal et al., "Exercise and Pharmacotherapy in the Treatment of Major Depressive Disorder," *Psychosomatic Medicine* 69 (August 2007): 587–96.

13. Irving Kirsch et al., "Initial Severity and Antidepressant Benefits: A Meta-Analysis of Data Submitted to the Food and Drug Administration," *PLoS Medicine*, Public Library of Science (August/September 2008).

14. Of note in this connection is *intuition medicine*, a new discipline developed under the guidance of Francesca McCartney, which has recently become a formalized area of professional training at the Academy of Intuition Medicine and Energy Medicine University, in Sausalito, California. The academy's PhD programs are certified by the State of California. See http://www.intuitionmedicine.com/academy/founder.htm.

15. Senator Tom Harkin, "Fighting Disease, and Remaking America as a Wellness Society," Senator Harkin's Official Senate Website, http://harkin.senate.gov/issue/healthcare.cfm.

16. Dean Ornish et al., "Changes in prostate gene expression in men undergoing an intensive nutrition and lifestyle intervention," *PNAS* 105, no. 24 (June 17, 2008): 8369–74.

17. The Institute for Health and Socio-Economic Policy is the research arm of the California Nurses Association and its national arm, the National Nurses Organizing Committee. The CNA/NNOC is a leading national advocate for health care reform. See the full report at http://www.calnurses.org/research/.

Chapter 8

1. See www.healthmedicinecenter.net.

Chapter 9

1. Donna Smith, "Big Insurance Shows Its Hand—or at Least Its Finger" (October 30, 2008), CommonDreams.org, http://www. commondreams.org/view/2008/10/30-6.

2. For more background on integral theory and the integral worldview, see Integral Institute, http://www.integralinstitute.org/.

3. Kenneth Thorpe, "The Obama Budget and Health Reform," *Huffington Post* (February 25, 2009).

4. Deepak Chopra et al., "Alternative Medicine Is Mainstream," *Wall Street Journal* (January 9, 2009).

5. Paul Krugman, "The Health Care Racket," *New York Times* (February 16, 2007).

6. Cathy Schoen et al., "In Chronic Condition: Experiences of Patients with Complex Health Care Needs, in Eight Countries, 2008," *Health Affairs* 28, no. 1 (2009): w1–w16.

7. Steffie Woolhandler, Oliver Fein, Mark Almberg, Physicians for a National Health Program, "Doctors to Candidates: Enact Single-Payer Health Reform" (October 6, 2008), PNHP.org.

8. See Senator Tom Harkin, "Iowa for Health Care Hosts Roundtable Discussion in Cedar Rapids in Iowa's 37th House District," http://www.iowaforhealthcare.org/. Accessed February 15, 2009.

9. Joe Conason, "Obama Pushes Universal Health Foes to the Margins," *New York Observer*, February 25, 2009.

10. FAIR, "FAIR Study: Media Blackout on Single-Payer Healthcare" (March 6, 2009), http://www.fair.org/index.php?page=3733.

11. Paul Krugman, "One Nation, Uninsured," *New York Times*, June 13, 2005.

12. Ronald T. Ackermann and Aaron E. Carroll, "Support for National Health Insurance among U.S. Physicians: A National Survey," *Annals of Internal Medicine* 139, issue 10 (November 18, 2003): 795–801.